MW01601070

Super Easy Mediterranean Diet Cookbook for Seniors

Evidence-Based Recipes with a 28-Day Meal Plan to Boost Energy, Improve Heart and Brain Health, and Support Strong, Healthy Aging

Helen Parker

Contents

INTRODUCTION

What Makes This Cookbook Different?

Aging doesn't mean giving up flavor, energy, or joy in the kitchen. In fact, the right food can help you feel stronger, think clearer, move easier and enjoy life more fully. This cookbook is built on that promise.

You won't find fad diets or complicated plans here. Instead, you'll find simple, delicious, research-backed recipes designed specifically for seniors. Every dish in this book is crafted to support your body's changing needs—without sacrificing taste, satisfaction, or ease of preparation.

Whether you're cooking for yourself, your partner, or sharing a meal with family, you'll discover food that's comforting, healing, and energizing. Meals that help your heart beat stronger, your mind stay sharp, and your joints feel a little looser each day.

This recipe book is a tool for aging well with dignity, vitality, and flavor.

What Is the Mediterranean Diet?

The Mediterranean diet is a way of eating and living that comes from the coastal regions of countries like Greece, Italy, and Spain. People there eat a variety of fresh, wholesome foods every day and enjoy meals slowly, often in the company of others.

This diet focuses on:

- Fruits and vegetables
- Whole grains
- Healthy fats like olive oil and nuts
- Lean proteins, especially fish and legumes
- Herbs and spices instead of salt
- Limited red meat and processed foods

And perhaps most importantly, it's flexible. It doesn't require perfection—just consistency, balance, and enjoyment.

Why It's Especially Powerful for Seniors?

As we get older, our metabolism slows down. Muscle mass decreases. Bones get weaker. And the risk of chronic illnesses like heart disease, type 2 diabetes, and memory loss increases.

That's why seniors need more than just any healthy diet—they need one that's:

- Rich in antioxidants to protect the brain
- High in anti-inflammatory foods to soothe joints
- Naturally full of fiber for digestive health
- Packed with healthy fats and lean proteins to support muscle and heart strength
- Soft and easy to chew, where needed

- Balanced, satisfying, and enjoyable

The Mediterranean diet meets all of these needs deliciously.

Backed by Science: Evidence-Based Health Benefits

This cookbook is built on decades of research from institutions like the Mayo Clinic, Harvard School of Public Health, and European Heart Journal. It draws on major clinical trials like:

- **The PREDIMED Study** – Found that seniors following the Mediterranean diet had a 30% lower risk of heart attacks and strokes.
- **The MIND Diet Study** – Showed reduced risk of Alzheimer's in older adults who combined Mediterranean and DASH eating habits.
- **Meta-Analyses** – Confirmed the diet's ability to improve insulin sensitivity, lower blood pressure, and reduce inflammation.

Every recipe in this book includes a quick evidence-based note about how it supports your heart, brain, bones, or digestion—so you always know what your food is doing for you.

The Role of Diet in Managing Aging-Related Conditions

Food is more than fuel. It's medicine and daily prevention. By focusing on the right foods, you can actively support your body's natural healing and resilience. This cookbook includes recipes that:

- Protect your heart with omega-3s, fiber, and antioxidants
- Boost memory and mental clarity with brain-healthy fats and anti-inflammatory produce
- Support strong bones with calcium, vitamin D, and protein
- Manage blood sugar and prevent type 2 diabetes through balanced carbs and healthy fats
- Improve digestion and reduce constipation with fiber-rich grains and vegetables
- Ease inflammation through turmeric, olive oil, and leafy greens

Each chapter is designed to be approachable, delicious, and functional—so that every meal supports not just your appetite, but your well-being.

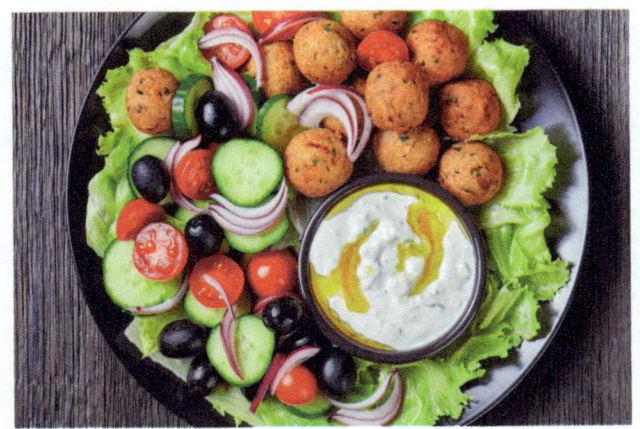

Nutrition & Wellness Over 60

Key Nutrients for Aging Gracefully

As we age, our bodies undergo changes that affect how we absorb and use nutrients. That's why seniors need more than just calories they need nutrient-dense foods that deliver maximum health benefits in every bite.

Here are the key nutrients older adults need most and how the Mediterranean diet naturally provides them:

- **Protein** – Helps preserve muscle mass, support healing, and maintain strength. Sources: eggs, legumes, fish, yogurt.
- **Calcium & Vitamin D** – Essential for bone density and preventing fractures. Sources: leafy greens, low-fat dairy, sardines, fortified plant milks.
- **Omega-3 Fatty Acids** – Reduce inflammation and support brain and heart health. Sources: salmon, walnuts, flaxseeds.
- **B Vitamins (especially B12)** – Vital for brain function, energy metabolism, and red blood cell production. Sources: eggs, poultry, fortified grains.
- **Fiber** – Aids digestion, regulates blood sugar, and lowers cholesterol. Sources: whole grains, fruits, vegetables, legumes.
- **Magnesium & Potassium** – Help manage blood pressure and support nerve and muscle function. Sources: bananas, spinach, nuts, whole grains.

The Mediterranean diet emphasizes all of these through natural, whole foods —making it one of the most nourishing eating patterns for people over 60.

Common Conditions the Mediterranean Diet Helps Prevent & Manage

Backed by decades of scientific research, the Mediterranean diet is a powerful tool in reducing the risk and even managing the progression of many chronic conditions common in older adults.

Heart Disease & High Blood Pressure

Numerous studies show that diets rich in healthy fats (like olive oil and fatty fish), fiber, and antioxidants help lower blood pressure, reduce bad cholesterol (LDL), and decrease inflammation. The PREDIMED Study (New England Journal of Medicine, 2013) found that seniors following a Mediterranean diet had up to a 30% lower risk of major cardiovascular events.

Cognitive Decline & Alzheimer's

The Mediterranean diet supports brain health through antioxidant-rich fruits and vegetables, omega-3s, and polyphenols. Research from the MIND diet (a Mediterranean-DASH hybrid) showed participants reduced their risk of Alzheimer's by up to 53% when closely following the diet (Rush University, 2015).

Type 2 Diabetes

Whole grains, legumes, and healthy fats slow down glucose absorption and improve insulin sensitivity.

A 2014 meta-analysis published in the American Journal of Clinical Nutrition found that the Mediterranean diet reduced the risk of developing type 2 diabetes by up to 19% and helped manage blood sugar levels in existing diabetics.

Osteoporosis & Bone Health

Bone strength relies on nutrients like calcium, vitamin D, magnesium, and protein—all abundant in Mediterranean foods. Leafy greens, dairy, legumes, and fish like sardines support skeletal health while anti-inflammatory properties reduce bone loss.

Arthritis & Inflammation

Chronic inflammation is a key driver of arthritis pain. Olive oil, berries, leafy greens, and fatty fish have been shown to reduce inflammatory markers like CRP. Studies in Arthritis Research & Therapy highlight improvements in joint stiffness and swelling among seniors following anti-inflammatory diets like this one.

Digestive Issues & Constipation

Slower digestion is common with age. The Mediterranean diet's high fiber content from fruits, vegetables, legumes, and whole grains supports gut health, reduces bloating, and promotes regularity.

Reading Labels & Portion Control for Seniors

Cooking from whole ingredients is ideal but grocery shopping still requires label literacy. Here's how seniors can quickly assess if a product supports their health:

- **Sodium:** Aim for less than 400–500 mg per meal
- **Added Sugar:** Keep as low as possible; avoid hidden sugars
- Fiber: Look for at least 3g per serving
- **Protein:** Target 10–20g per meal depending on activity level
- **Saturated Fat:** Keep under 3g per serving

Smart Portioning Tips:

- Use smaller plates to naturally control portions
- Fill half the plate with vegetables, a quarter with lean protein, and a quarter with whole grains
- Listen to hunger cues instead of external portion sizes
- Store leftovers in single-serve containers for easy reheating

Kitchen Tools & Safety Tips for Seniors

Cooking should be safe and stress-free. Consider these tips for maintaining comfort and safety in the kitchen:

- Use non-slip mats and grip-handled tools to reduce strain
- Invest in lightweight pans and easy-open jars

- Keep a stool or chair nearby for rest during prep
- Store frequently used items at waist level to avoid bending or reaching
- Use a timer or smart speaker to prevent overcooking or forgetfulness

Accessible tools and organized prep help ensure that cooking stays an enjoyable and health-supportive— part of daily life.

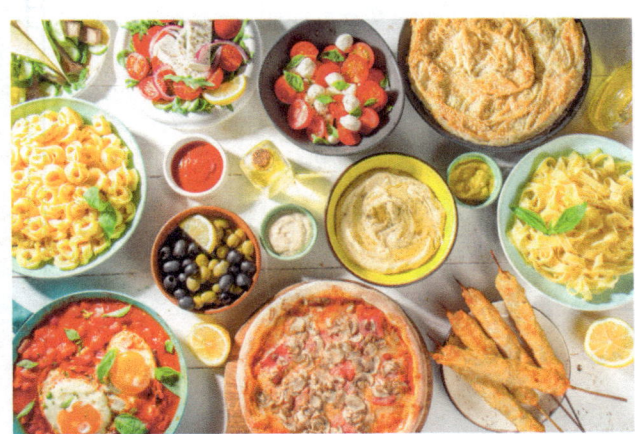

The Recipies

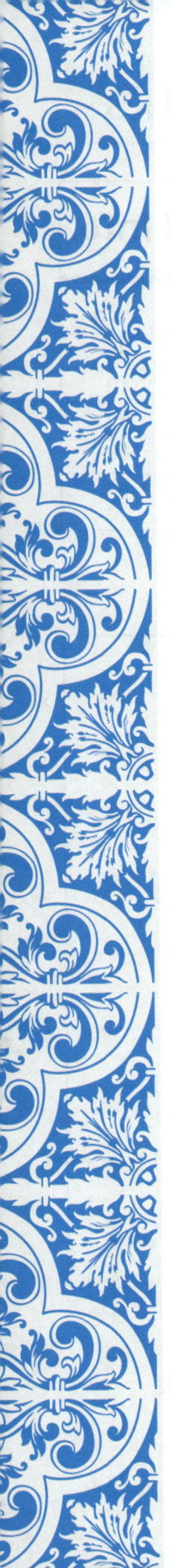

Energizing Breakfasts

Greek Yogurt Parfait with Berries & Walnuts

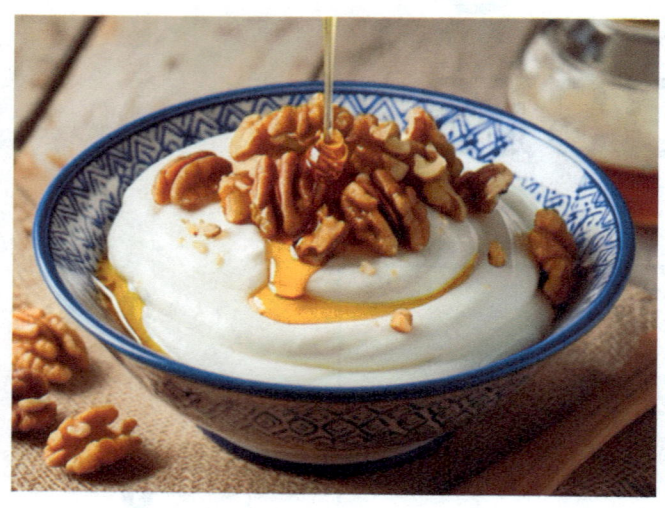

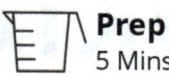 **Prep**
5 Mins

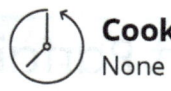 **Cook**
None

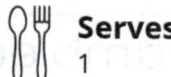 **Serves**
1

Nutritional Info.
(approx. per serving)

Calories:	210
Fiber(g):	3
Protein(g):	12
Healthy Fats(g):	8
Sodium(mg):	40
Carbs(g):	18

Ingredients

- ¾ cup plain Greek yogurt (unsweetened, full-fat or low-fat)
- ½ cup fresh mixed berries (blueberries, strawberries, raspberries)
- 1 tbsp chopped walnuts
- 1 tsp honey (optional)
- ½ tsp ground cinnamon (optional)

Instructions

- Spoon Greek yogurt into a bowl or parfait glass.
- Top with mixed berries.
- Sprinkle with chopped walnuts.
- Drizzle honey and dust with cinnamon, if using.
- Serve immediately.

Evidence-Based Health Note

Greek yogurt is rich in protein and calcium for bone strength. Berries provide antioxidants that support brain health.

Olive Oil Scrambled Eggs with Spinach

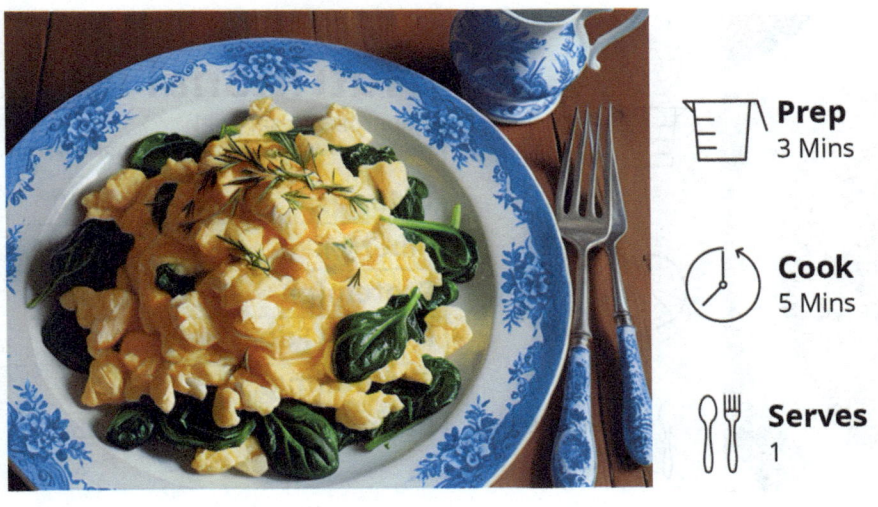

Prep
3 Mins

Cook
5 Mins

Serves
1

Nutritional Info. (approx. per serving)	
Calories:	240
Fiber(g):	1.5
Protein(g):	14
Healthy Fats(g):	17
Sodium(mg):	210
Carbs(g):	2

Ingredients

- 2 large eggs
- 1 tsp extra virgin olive oil
- ½ cup fresh spinach, chopped
- Salt and black pepper to taste
- Pinch of turmeric (optional, for joint health)

Instructions

- Crack eggs into a bowl, add a pinch of salt, pepper, and turmeric. Beat lightly.
- Heat olive oil in a nonstick pan over medium heat.
- Add chopped spinach and sauté for 1 minute until slightly wilted.
- Pour in the eggs. Stir gently and cook for 2–3 minutes, until softly scrambled.
- Serve warm with whole-grain toast if desired.

Evidence-Based Health Note

Eggs offer high-quality protein for muscle maintenance. Spinach adds lutein and folate, supporting eye and cognitive health.

Oatmeal with Chia Seeds and Almonds

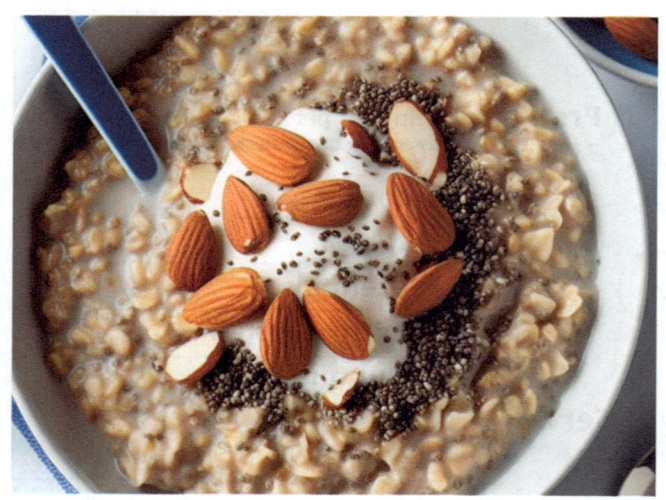

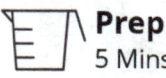 **Prep**
5 Mins

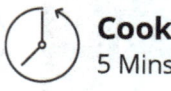 **Cook**
5 Mins

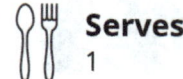 **Serves**
1

Nutritional Info.
(approx. per serving)

Calories:	280
Fiber(g):	5
Protein(g):	8
Healthy Fats(g):	10
Sodium(mg):	5
Carbs(g):	35

Ingredients

- ½ cup rolled oats
- 1 cup water or low-fat milk
- 1 tbsp chia seeds
- 1 tbsp sliced almonds
- 1 tsp honey (optional)
- ¼ tsp cinnamon

Instructions

- In a small pot, bring the water or milk to a boil.
- Stir in oats and reduce to a simmer for 4–5 minutes, stirring occasionally.
- Once thickened, remove from heat and stir in chia seeds and cinnamon.
- Pour into a bowl and top with almonds and honey if desired.
- Serve warm.

Evidence-Based Health Note

Oats provide soluble fiber that lowers cholesterol. Chia seeds are rich in omega-3s and promote joint and heart health.

Avocado Toast on Whole-Grain Bread

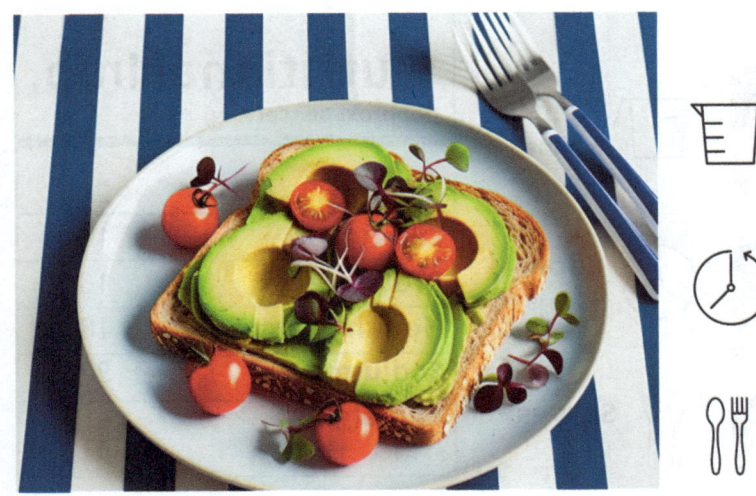

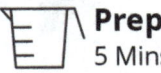
Prep
5 Mins

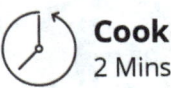
Cook
2 Mins

Serves
1

Nutritional Info.	
(approx. per serving)	
Calories:	300
Fiber(g):	6
Protein(g):	7
Healthy Fats(g):	16
Sodium(mg):	180
Carbs(g):	28

Ingredients

- 1 slice whole-grain bread
- ½ ripe avocado
- 1 tsp extra virgin olive oil
- A squeeze of lemon juice
- A pinch of salt and black pepper
- Optional toppings: sliced radish, cherry tomatoes, or red pepper flakes

Instructions

- Toast the whole-grain bread to your desired crispness.
- In a bowl, mash the avocado with lemon juice, salt, and pepper.
- Spread the avocado mash evenly over the toast.
- Drizzle with olive oil.
- Add optional toppings if desired. Serve immediately.

Evidence-Based Health Note

Avocados are high in heart-healthy monounsaturated fats. Whole-grain bread offers fiber for digestion and blood sugar control.

Tomato & Feta Omelet

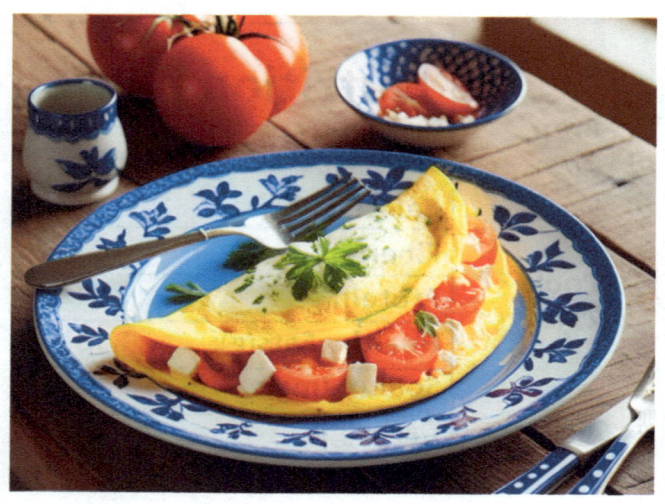

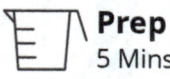
Prep
5 Mins

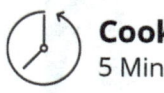
Cook
5 Mins

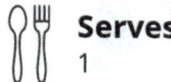
Serves
1

Nutritional Info.
(approx. per serving)

Calories:	270
Fiber(g):	1
Protein(g):	16
Healthy Fats(g):	18
Sodium(mg):	320
Carbs(g):	4

Ingredients

- 2 large eggs
- ¼ cup crumbled feta cheese
- ½ tomato, diced
- 1 tsp olive oil
- Pinch of oregano
- Salt and pepper to taste

Instructions

- Beat eggs in a bowl with salt, pepper, and oregano.
- Heat olive oil in a nonstick pan over medium heat.
- Pour in eggs and cook for 1–2 minutes.
- Add tomato and feta on one half.
- Fold omelet and cook another 2 minutes until set.
- Serve hot.

Evidence-Based Health Note

Eggs support brain and muscle function. Tomatoes deliver lycopene, which may reduce heart disease risk.

Mediterranean Breakfast Quinoa Bowl

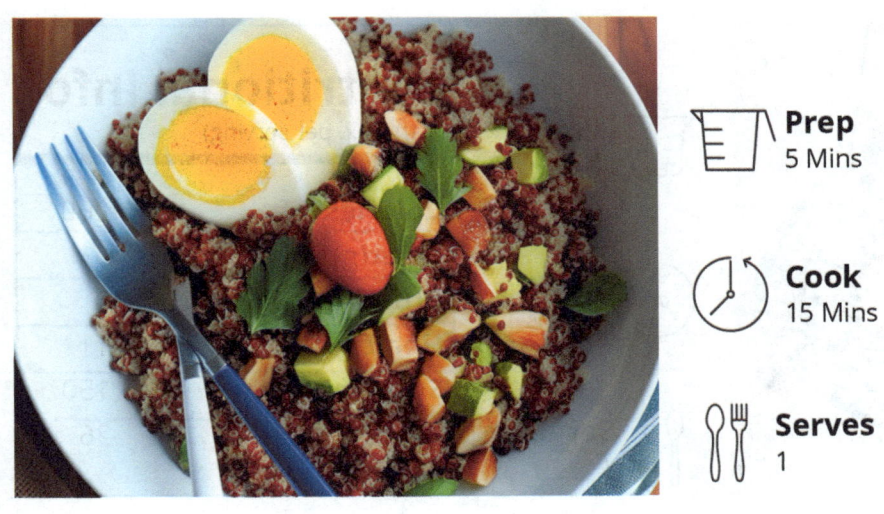

Prep
5 Mins

Cook
15 Mins

Serves
1

Nutritional Info.	
(approx. per serving)	
Calories:	310
Fiber(g):	4
Protein(g):	12
Healthy Fats(g):	14
Sodium(mg):	200
Carbs(g):	34

Ingredients

- ½ cup cooked quinoa
- ¼ avocado, diced
- 1 boiled egg, sliced
- 2 tbsp hummus
- ¼ cup chopped cucumber
- 1 tsp olive oil
- Pinch of paprika

Instructions

- Place cooked quinoa in a bowl.
- Arrange avocado, egg, cucumber, and hummus on top.
- Drizzle with olive oil and sprinkle with paprika.
- Serve warm or at room temperature.

Evidence-Based Health Note

Quinoa offers complete protein and fiber. Avocado and olive oil provide fats that reduce inflammation and support heart health.

Ricotta Toast with Strawberries & Basil

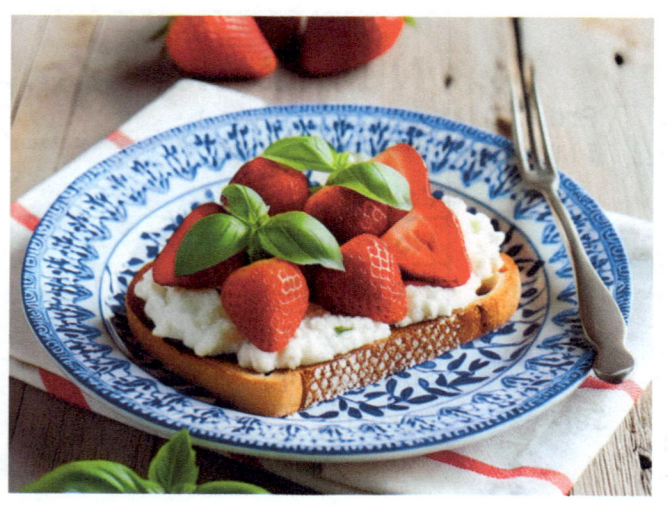

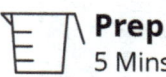 **Prep**
5 Mins

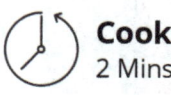 **Cook**
2 Mins

Serves
1

Nutritional Info.
(approx. per serving)

Calories:	260
Fiber(g):	3
Protein(g):	9
Healthy Fats(g):	11
Sodium(mg):	150
Carbs(g):	26

Ingredients

- 1 slice whole-grain bread
- ¼ cup ricotta cheese
- 2–3 strawberries, sliced
- 2–3 fresh basil leaves
- 1 tsp honey (optional)

Instructions

- Toast the bread to your liking.
- Spread ricotta evenly on toast.
- Top with sliced strawberries and torn basil.
- Drizzle with honey if desired.
- Serve immediately.

Evidence-Based Health Note

Ricotta supplies calcium for bone strength. Strawberries are packed with vitamin C and brain-protective antioxidants.

Spinach & Mushroom Breakfast Wrap

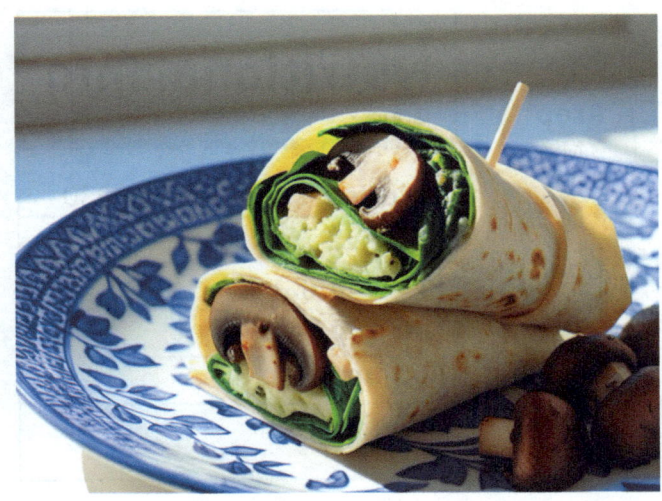

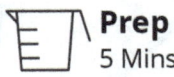
Prep
5 Mins

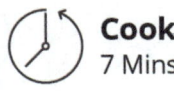
Cook
7 Mins

Serves
1

Nutritional Info.
(approx. per serving)

Calories:	290
Fiber(g):	4
Protein(g):	13
Healthy Fats(g):	12
Sodium(mg):	270
Carbs(g):	27

Ingredients

- 1 whole-grain tortilla
- 1 egg
- ¼ cup sliced mushrooms
- ½ cup baby spinach
- 1 tsp olive oil
- Salt & pepper to taste

Instructions

- Heat olive oil in a pan over medium heat.
- Sauté mushrooms for 2–3 minutes, then add spinach and cook until wilted.
- Push to one side and scramble the egg on the other side.
- Combine and transfer to tortilla.
- Wrap tightly and serve warm.

Evidence-Based Health Note

Spinach and mushrooms provide fiber and anti-inflammatory nutrients. Eggs add protein for sustained energy.

Banana Nut Smoothie with Flaxseed

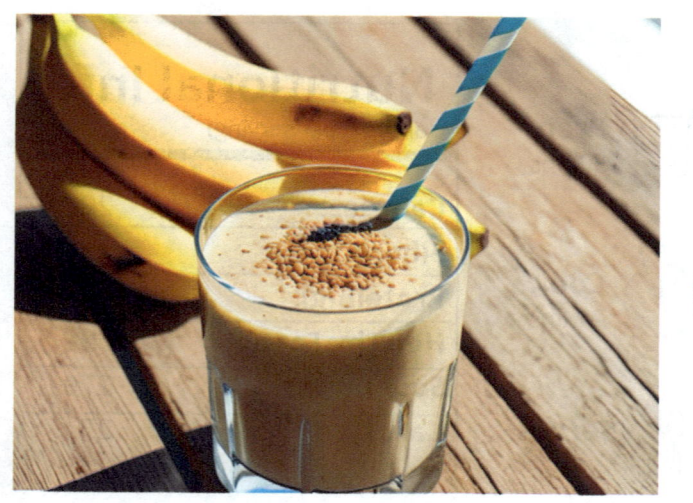

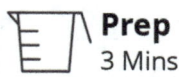
Prep
3 Mins

Cook
None

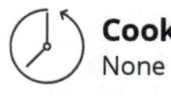
Serves
1 glass

Nutritional Info.
(approx. per serving)

Calories:	230
Fiber(g):	4
Protein(g):	10
Healthy Fats(g):	9
Sodium(mg):	6
Carbs(g):	25

Ingredients

- 1 banana
- ¾ cup unsweetened almond milk
- 1 tbsp ground flaxseed
- 1 tbsp peanut or almond butter
- 2–3 ice cubes

Instructions

- Add all ingredients to a blender.
- Blend until smooth.
- Serve immediately.

Evidence-Based Health Note

Flaxseed provides omega-3s and fiber for heart and joint support. Bananas offer potassium to regulate blood pressure.

Cottage Cheese with Olives & Cherry Tomatoes

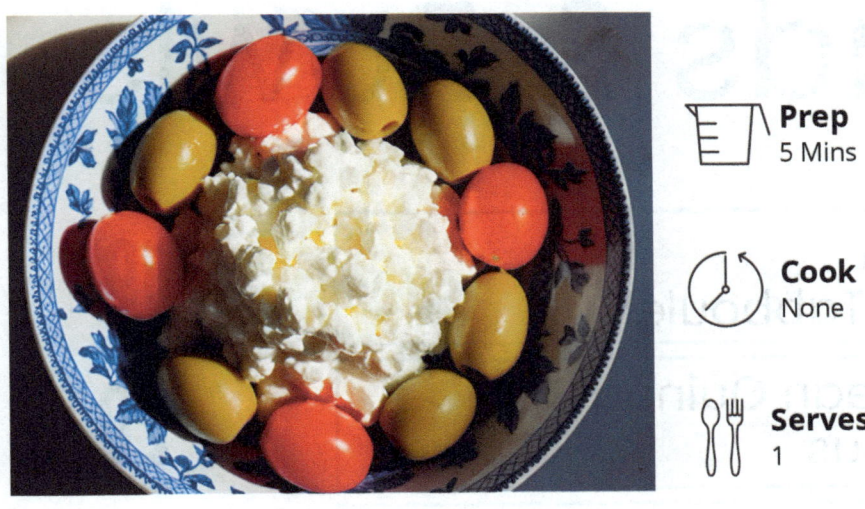

Prep
5 Mins

Cook
None

Serves
1

Nutritional Info.
(approx. per serving)

Calories:	200
Fiber(g):	2
Protein(g):	15
Healthy Fats(g):	10
Sodium(mg):	250
Carbs(g):	6

Ingredients

- ½ cup low-fat cottage cheese
- 5–6 cherry tomatoes, halved
- 4–5 pitted Kalamata olives, sliced
- 1 tsp extra virgin olive oil
- A pinch of black pepper
- Optional: sprinkle of dried oregano or fresh basil leaves

Instructions

- Spoon the cottage cheese into a small bowl.
- Add the halved cherry tomatoes and sliced olives on top.
- Drizzle with olive oil.
- Sprinkle with pepper and herbs if using.
- Serve immediately, optionally with whole-grain crackers.

Evidence-Based Health Note

Cottage cheese is high in protein for muscle preservation. Olives add heart-healthy fats and antioxidants.

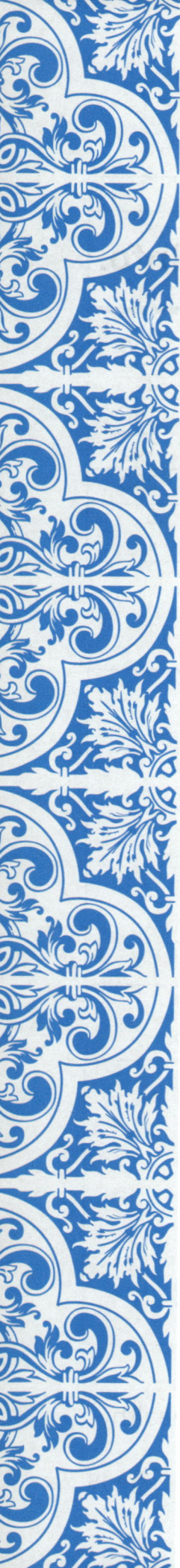

Nourishing Salads & Bowls

Chickpea & Cucumber Tabbouleh

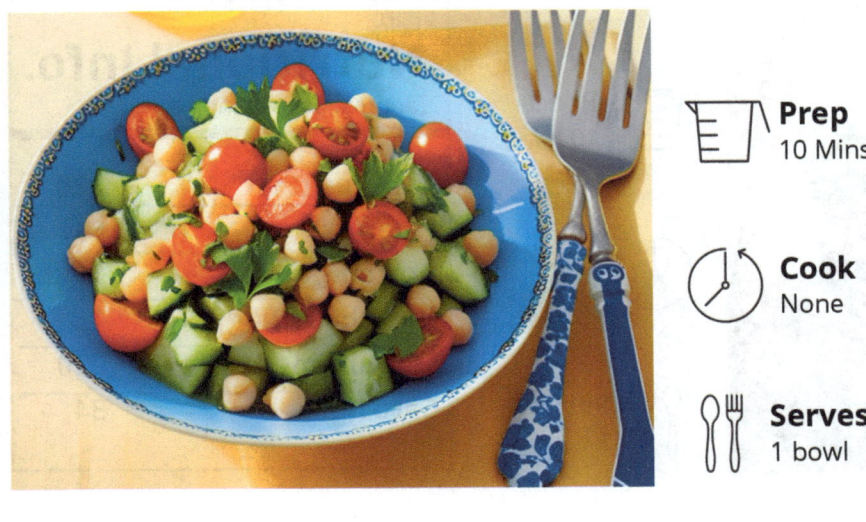

Prep
10 Mins

Cook
None

Serves
1 bowl

Nutritional Info.
(approx. per serving)

Calories:	250
Fiber(g):	6
Protein(g):	9
Healthy Fats(g):	8
Sodium(mg):	150
Carbs(g):	30

Ingredients

- ½ cup cooked chickpeas (or canned, rinsed)
- ½ cup chopped cucumber
- ¼ cup chopped parsley
- 2 tbsp diced red onion
- Juice of ½ lemon
- 1 tsp olive oil
- Salt and pepper to taste

Instructions

- Combine chickpeas, cucumber, parsley, and onion in a bowl.
- Drizzle with olive oil and lemon juice.
- Season with salt and pepper.
- Mix gently and serve chilled.

Evidence-Based Health Note

Chickpeas provide plant-based protein and fiber, which support heart health and digestion.

Mediterranean Quinoa Bowl with Hummus

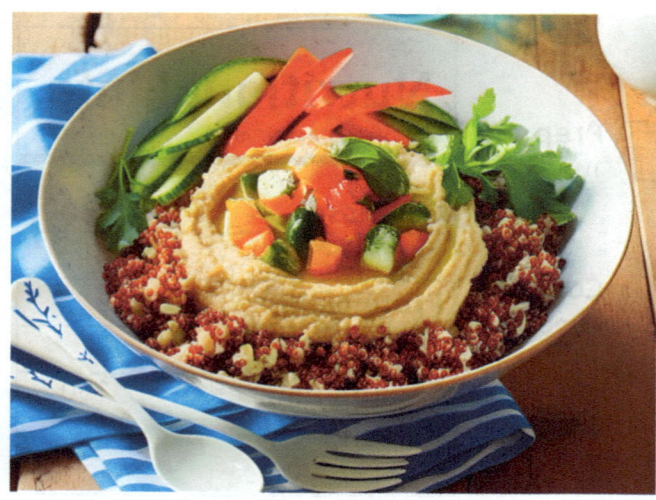

Prep
10 Mins

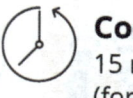
Cook
15 mins
(for quinoa)

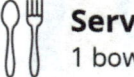
Serves
1 bowl

Nutritional Info.
(approx. per serving)

Calories:	320
Fiber(g):	5
Protein(g):	11
Healthy Fats(g):	13
Sodium(mg):	220
Carbs(g):	34

Ingredients

- ½ cup cooked quinoa
- ¼ cup cherry tomatoes, halved
- ¼ avocado, sliced
- ¼ cup chopped cucumber
- 2 tbsp hummus
- 1 tsp olive oil
- Pinch of za'atar or paprika (optional)

Instructions

- Place quinoa in a bowl.
- Arrange tomatoes, avocado, and cucumber on top.
- Add a scoop of hummus.
- Drizzle with olive oil and sprinkle seasoning if using.
- Serve immediately or chilled.

Evidence-Based Health Note

Quinoa and hummus deliver fiber and healthy fats that stabilize blood sugar and reduce inflammation.

Greek Salad with Olive Oil & Feta

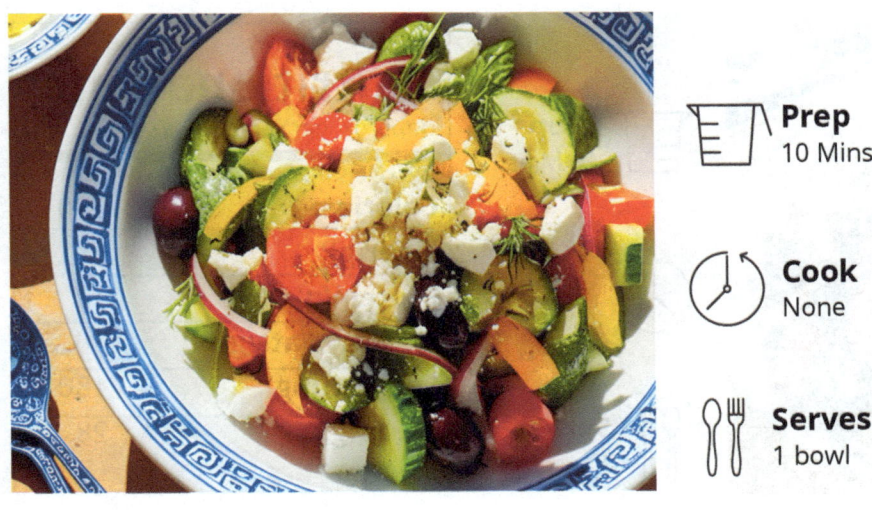

Prep
10 Mins

Cook
None

Serves
1 bowl

Nutritional Info.
(approx. per serving)

Calories:	210
Fiber(g):	3
Protein(g):	6
Healthy Fats(g):	14
Sodium(mg):	280
Carbs(g):	10

Ingredients

- ½ cup chopped cucumber
- ¼ cup cherry tomatoes, halved
- 2 tbsp sliced red onion
- ¼ cup diced feta cheese
- 4–5 olives, sliced
- 1 tsp olive oil
- Dash of oregano

Instructions

- Combine vegetables in a bowl.
- Add feta and olives.
- Drizzle with olive oil and sprinkle oregano.
- Toss gently and serve.

Evidence-Based Health Note

Feta adds calcium for bone strength. Olive oil contains antioxidants that support heart health.

Lentil & Roasted Veggie Salad

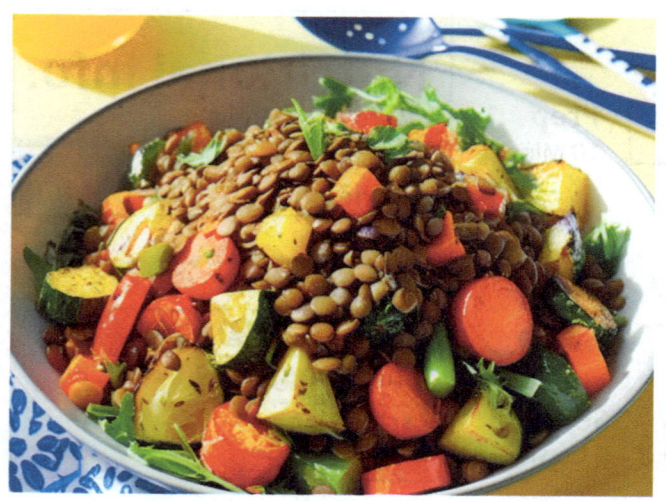

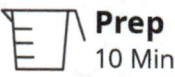 **Prep**
10 Mins

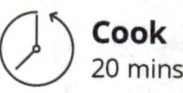 **Cook**
20 mins

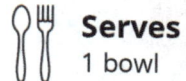 **Serves**
1 bowl

Nutritional Info.
(approx. per serving)

Calories:	270
Fiber(g):	7
Protein(g):	12
Healthy Fats(g):	10
Sodium(mg):	180
Carbs(g):	28

Ingredients

- ½ cup cooked lentils
- ¼ cup roasted carrots
- ¼ cup roasted bell peppers
- 1 tbsp chopped parsley
- 1 tsp olive oil
- 1 tsp lemon juice
- Salt and pepper

Instructions

- Combine lentils and roasted vegetables in a bowl.
- Add parsley.
- Drizzle with olive oil and lemon juice.
- Toss and serve warm or chilled.

Evidence-Based Health Note

Lentils offer cholesterol-lowering fiber. Roasted vegetables provide antioxidants that fight inflammation.

Tuna & White Bean Salad

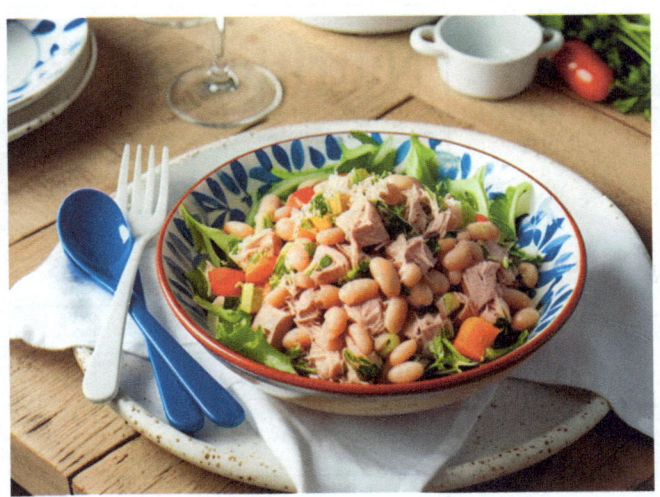

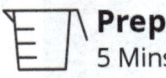 **Prep**
5 Mins

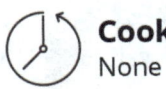 **Cook**
None

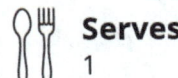 **Serves**
1

Nutritional Info.
(approx. per serving)

Calories:	300
Fiber(g):	5
Protein(g):	20
Healthy Fats(g):	13
Sodium(mg):	260
Carbs(g):	18

Ingredients

- ½ cup canned white beans, rinsed
- ¼ cup canned tuna in olive oil, drained
- 1 tbsp chopped parsley
- 1 tsp lemon juice
- Salt and pepper

Instructions

- Mix beans, tuna, and parsley in a bowl.
- Drizzle lemon juice over.
- Add salt and pepper to taste.
- Serve chilled.

Evidence-Based Health Note

Tuna provides omega-3s for heart and brain health. White beans add fiber and plant-based protein.

Caprese Salad with Balsamic Glaze

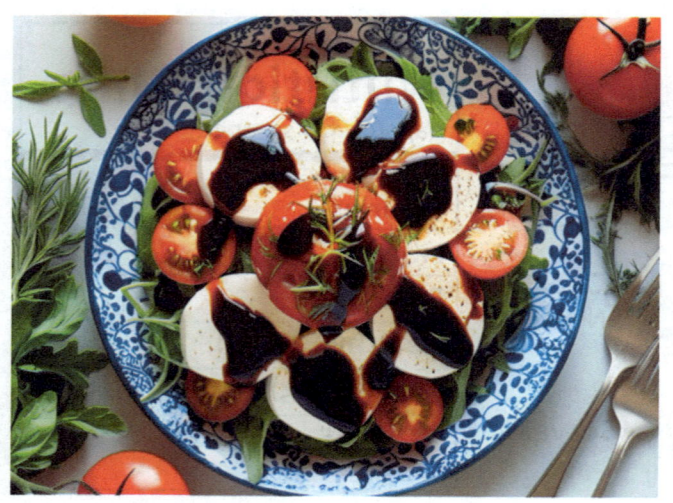

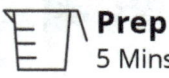 **Prep**
5 Mins

Cook
None

Serves
1

Nutritional Info.	
(approx. per serving)	
Calories:	200
Fiber(g):	1
Protein(g):	9
Healthy Fats(g):	12
Sodium(mg):	150
Carbs(g):	10

Ingredients

- 3 slices fresh mozzarella
- 3 slices tomato
- 3–4 fresh basil leaves
- 1 tsp olive oil
- ½ tsp balsamic glaze

Instructions

- Layer tomato and mozzarella slices alternately.
- Top with basil leaves.
- Drizzle olive oil and balsamic glaze.
- Serve fresh.

Evidence-Based Health Note

Tomatoes offer lycopene, linked to lower heart disease risk. Mozzarella provides calcium for bone health.

Roasted Beet & Walnut Salad

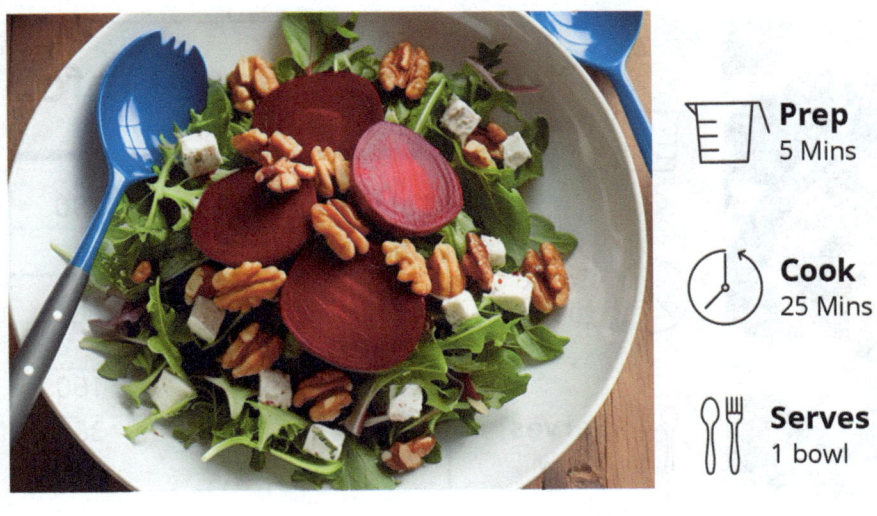

Prep
5 Mins

Cook
25 Mins

Serves
1 bowl

Nutritional Info.
(approx. per serving)

Calories:	240
Fiber(g):	4
Protein(g):	5
Healthy Fats(g):	11
Sodium(mg):	140
Carbs(g):	20

Ingredients

- ½ cup cooked or roasted beets, diced
- 1 tbsp chopped walnuts
- 1 tbsp crumbled feta (optional)
- 1 tsp olive oil
- 1 tsp lemon juice
- Pinch of salt

Instructions

- Combine beets, walnuts, and feta in a bowl.
- Drizzle olive oil and lemon juice.
- Toss lightly and serve.

Evidence-Based Health Note

Beets support blood pressure regulation. Walnuts are rich in omega-3s that promote brain health.

Farro Salad with Herbs & Lemon

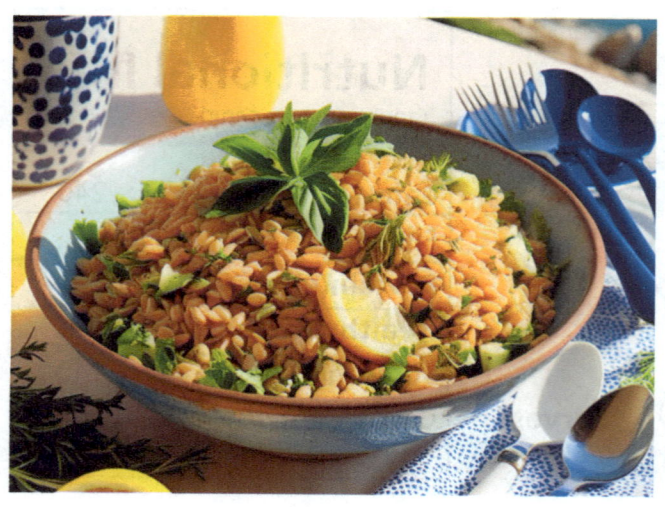

 **Prep**
10 Mins

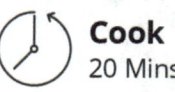 **Cook**
20 Mins

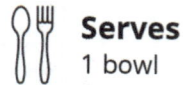 **Serves**
1 bowl

Nutritional Info.
(approx. per serving)

Calories:	290
Fiber(g):	5
Protein(g):	10
Healthy Fats(g):	9
Sodium(mg):	160
Carbs(g):	36

Ingredients

- ½ cup cooked farro
- 1 tbsp chopped mint or parsley
- ¼ cup chopped cucumber
- 1 tsp olive oil
- 1 tsp lemon zest and juice
- Salt and pepper

Instructions

- Mix cooked farro, cucumber, and herbs in a bowl.
- Add lemon zest, juice, olive oil, salt, and pepper.
- Toss and serve warm or chilled.

Evidence-Based Health Note

Farro is a whole grain high in magnesium and fiber, supporting heart and digestive health.

Arugula Salad with Orange & Almonds

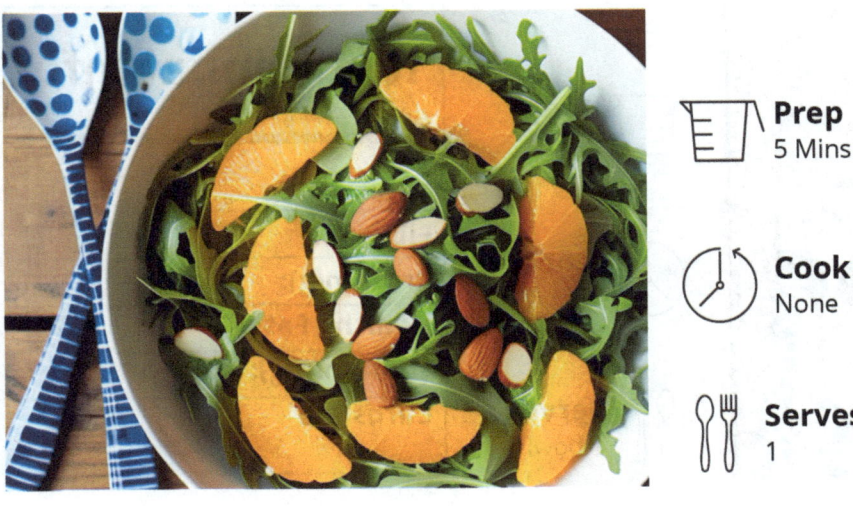

Prep
5 Mins

Cook
None

Serves
1

Nutritional Info.
(approx. per serving)

Calories:	220
Fiber(g):	3
Protein(g):	6
Healthy Fats(g):	11
Sodium(mg):	120
Carbs(g):	18

Ingredients

- 1 cup baby arugula
- ½ orange, peeled and sliced
- 1 tbsp sliced almonds
- 1 tsp olive oil
- Splash of orange juice

Instructions

- Place arugula in a bowl.
- Top with orange slices and almonds.
- Drizzle olive oil and juice.
- Toss lightly and serve.

Evidence-Based Health Note

Arugula is rich in bone-supporting vitamin K. Oranges add vitamin C for immune and joint health.

Spiced Chickpea Spinach Salad

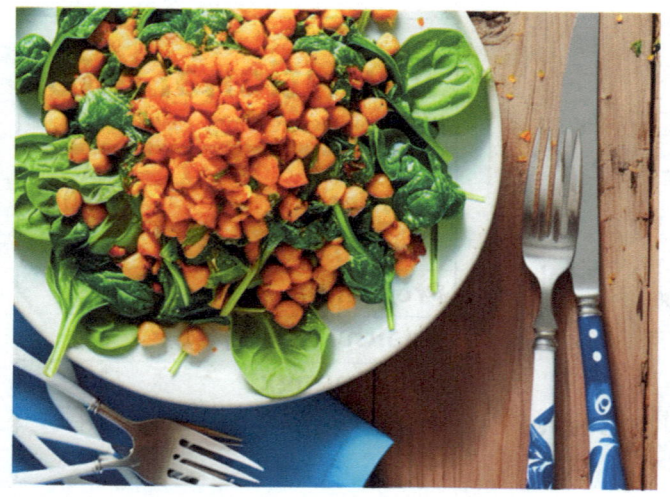

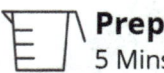 **Prep**
5 Mins

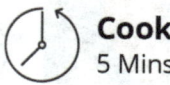 **Cook**
5 Mins

Serves
1 bowl

Nutritional Info.
(approx. per serving)

Calories:	260
Fiber(g):	6
Protein(g):	10
Healthy Fats(g):	10
Sodium(mg):	200
Carbs(g):	24

Ingredients

- ½ cup canned chickpeas, rinsed
- ½ cup fresh spinach
- 1 tsp olive oil
- ¼ tsp cumin
- ¼ tsp paprika
- Pinch of salt

Instructions

- Heat olive oil in a pan.
- Add chickpeas and spices, sauté for 3 minutes.
- Toss with fresh spinach until slightly wilted.
- Serve warm or room temperature.

Evidence-Based Health Note

Chickpeas provide protein and fiber. Spinach adds folate and antioxidants for cognitive health.

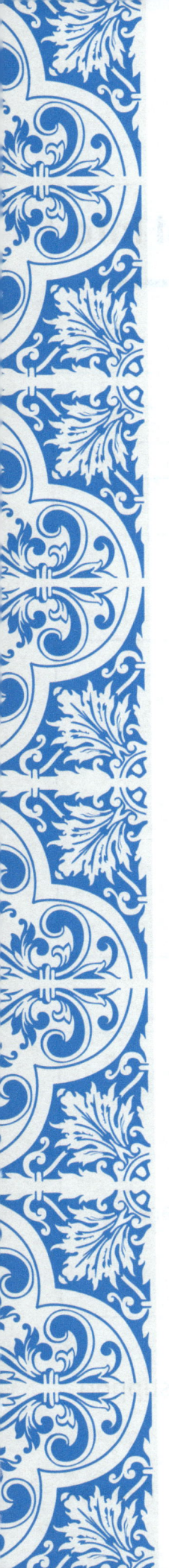

Comforting Soups & Stews

Lentil & Tomato Stew

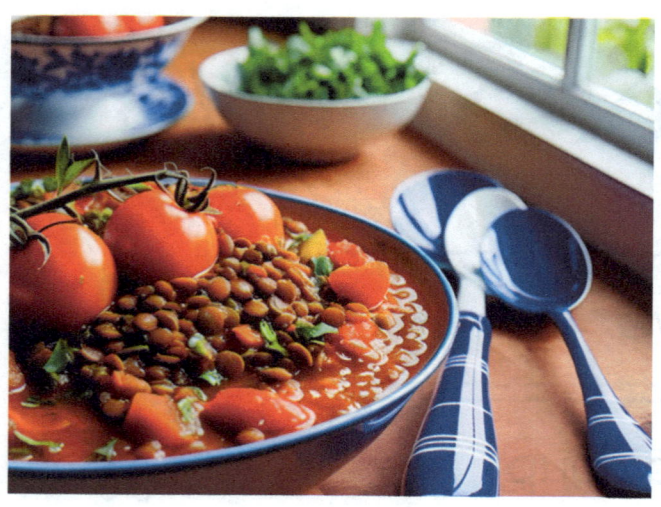

Prep
10 Mins

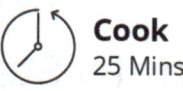
Cook
25 Mins

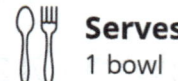
Serves
1 bowl

Nutritional Info.
(approx. per serving)

Calories:	280
Fiber(g):	8
Protein(g):	13
Healthy Fats(g):	7
Sodium(mg):	240
Carbs(g):	32

Ingredients

- ½ cup dried lentils (or 1 cup cooked)
- 1 cup chopped tomatoes (fresh or canned)
- ½ cup chopped onion
- 1 garlic clove, minced
- 1 tsp olive oil
- 1 cup low-sodium vegetable broth
- ½ tsp cumin
- Salt and pepper to taste

Instructions

- Heat olive oil in a pot over medium heat.
- Sauté onion and garlic for 3–4 minutes.
- Add tomatoes and cook for 2 more minutes.
- Add lentils, broth, cumin, salt, and pepper.
- Bring to a boil, reduce to simmer, and cook for 20–25 minutes or until lentils are soft.
- Serve warm.

Evidence-Based Health Note

Lentils are rich in fiber and plant protein, which help lower cholesterol and support heart health.

Lemon Chicken Orzo Soup

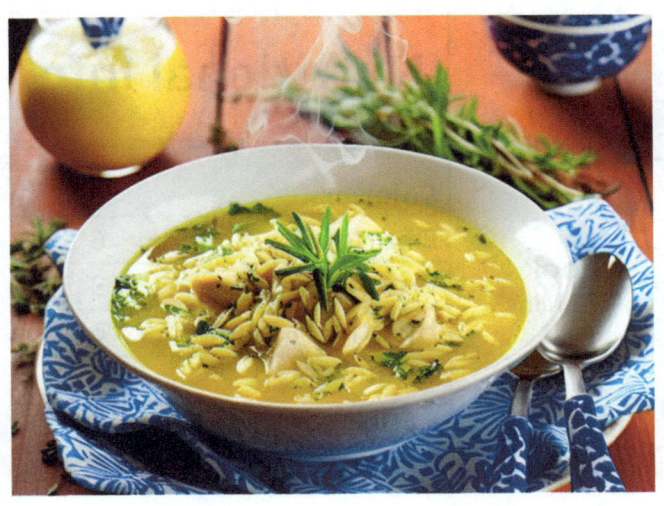

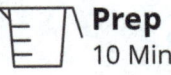 **Prep**
10 Mins

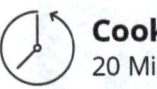 **Cook**
20 Mins

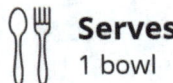 **Serves**
1 bowl

Nutritional Info.
(approx. per serving)

Calories:	260
Fiber(g):	2
Protein(g):	20
Healthy Fats(g):	8
Sodium(mg):	280
Carbs(g):	18

Ingredients

- ½ cup shredded cooked chicken
- 2 tbsp orzo pasta
- 1 cup low-sodium chicken broth
- ¼ cup chopped carrots
- 1 tbsp lemon juice
- 1 tsp olive oil
- Salt and pepper to taste

Instructions

- Heat olive oil in a saucepan and sauté carrots for 2–3 minutes.
- Add chicken broth and bring to a boil.
- Stir in orzo and cook for 10–12 minutes until tender.
- Add chicken and simmer for 5 more minutes.
- Stir in lemon juice, salt, and pepper. Serve hot.

Evidence-Based Health Note

Chicken provides lean protein for muscle maintenance. Lemon adds vitamin C, supporting immunity and digestion.

Minestrone with White Beans

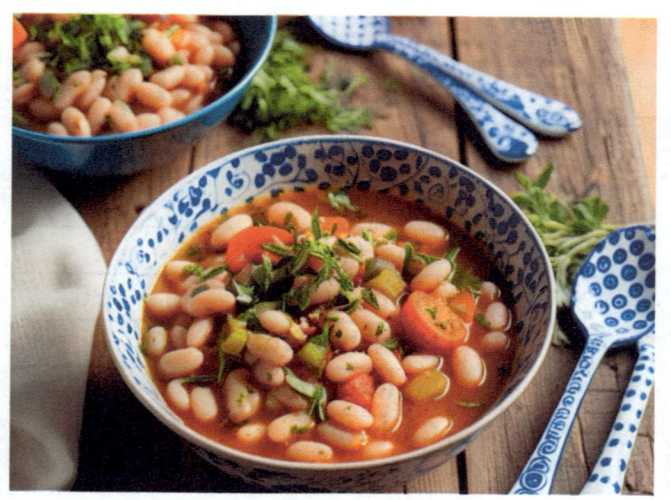

Prep
10 Mins

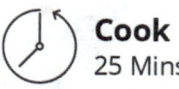
Cook
25 Mins

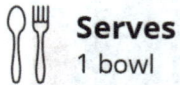
Serves
1 bowl

Nutritional Info.
(approx. per serving)

Calories:	230
Fiber(g):	6
Protein(g):	9
Healthy Fats(g):	6
Sodium(mg):	250
Carbs(g):	30

Ingredients

- ½ cup white beans (canned, rinsed)
- ½ cup chopped mixed vegetables (zucchini, carrots, celery)
- 1 cup vegetable broth
- ¼ cup canned diced tomatoes
- ¼ tsp Italian seasoning
- 1 tsp olive oil
- Salt to taste

Instructions

- In a pot, heat olive oil and sauté veggies for 5 minutes.
- Add tomatoes, beans, broth, and seasoning.
- Simmer uncovered for 20 minutes.
- Adjust salt to taste and serve warm.

Evidence-Based Health Note

White beans provide fiber and folate for heart and brain health. Vegetables deliver antioxidants for inflammation control.

Greek Egg-Lemon Soup (Avgolemono)

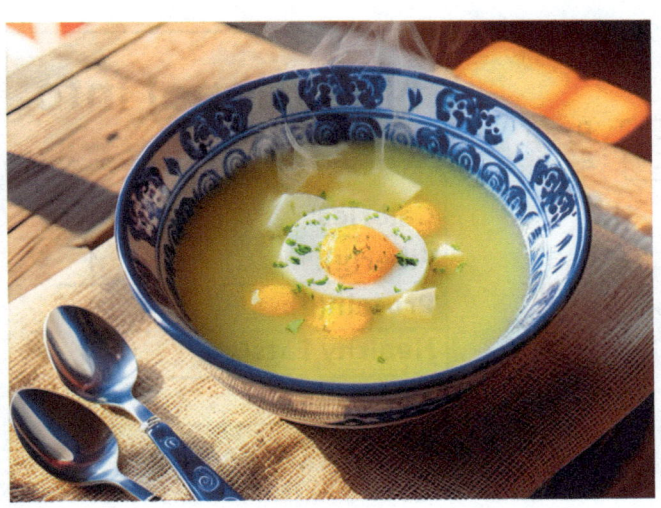

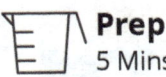 **Prep**
5 Mins

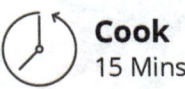 **Cook**
15 Mins

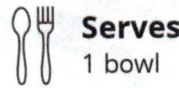 **Serves**
1 bowl

Nutritional Info.
(approx. per serving)

Calories:	240
Fiber(g):	1
Protein(g):	11
Healthy Fats(g):	10
Sodium(mg):	2601
Carbs(g):	16

Ingredients

- 1 egg
- 1 tbsp lemon juice
- 2 tbsp orzo or rice
- 1 cup chicken or vegetable broth
- Salt and pepper to taste

Instructions

- Cook orzo/rice in broth until tender.
- In a bowl, whisk egg and lemon juice together.
- Slowly add ½ cup hot broth into the egg mix while whisking.
- Return mixture to the pot and stir gently (do not boil).
- Season with salt and pepper and serve.

Evidence-Based Health Note

Eggs provide protein and B12 for brain health. Lemon and broth offer hydration and digestive support.

Roasted Red Pepper & Tomato Soup

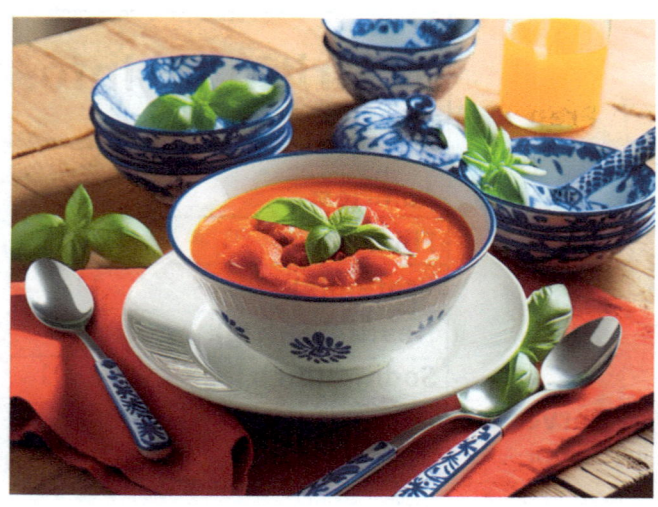

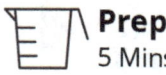 **Prep**
5 Mins

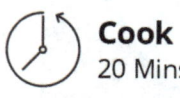 **Cook**
20 Mins

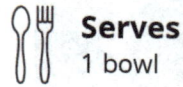 **Serves**
1 bowl

Nutritional Info.
(approx. per serving)

Calories:	190
Fiber(g):	4
Protein(g):	4
Healthy Fats(g):	7
Sodium(mg):	220
Carbs(g):	20

Ingredients

- 1 roasted red pepper (jarred or fresh)
- 1 cup chopped tomatoes
- ½ cup onion
- 1 garlic clove
- 1 tsp olive oil
- 1 cup vegetable broth
- Salt and pepper

Instructions

- Sauté onion and garlic in olive oil until soft.
- Add red pepper, tomatoes, and broth.
- Simmer for 15 minutes.
- Blend until smooth and season to taste.

Evidence-Based Health Note

Tomatoes and red peppers are rich in lycopene and vitamin C, both linked to heart and immune health.

Chickpea & Spinach Stew

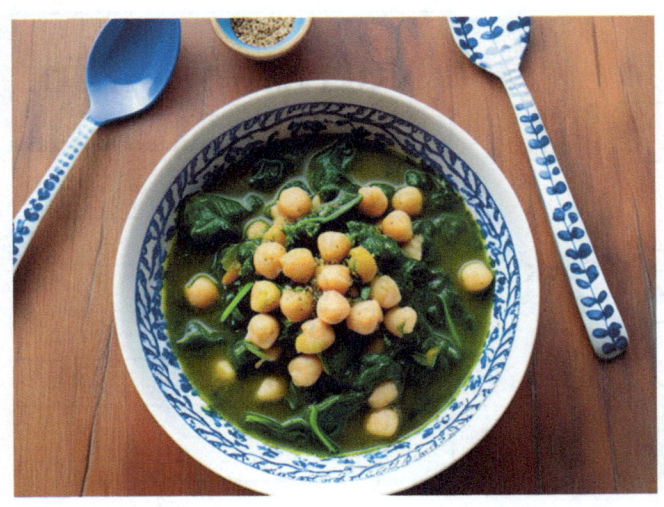

 **Prep**
10 Mins

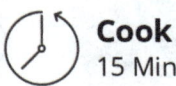 **Cook**
15 Mins

Serves
1 bowl

Nutritional Info.
(approx. per serving)

Calories:	270
Fiber(g):	7
Protein(g):	12
Healthy Fats(g):	9
Sodium(mg):	240
Carbs(g):	28

Ingredients

- ½ cup canned chickpeas
- 1 cup baby spinach
- ½ cup chopped tomatoes
- 1 garlic clove
- 1 tsp olive oil
- 1 cup vegetable broth
- Paprika or cumin (optional)

Instructions

- Heat oil and sauté garlic and tomatoes.
- Add chickpeas and broth, simmer for 10 minutes.
- Stir in spinach and cook until wilted.
- Season and serve.

Evidence-Based Health Note

Chickpeas provide plant protein and fiber. Spinach adds folate and antioxidants for brain and heart support.

Tuscan White Bean Soup

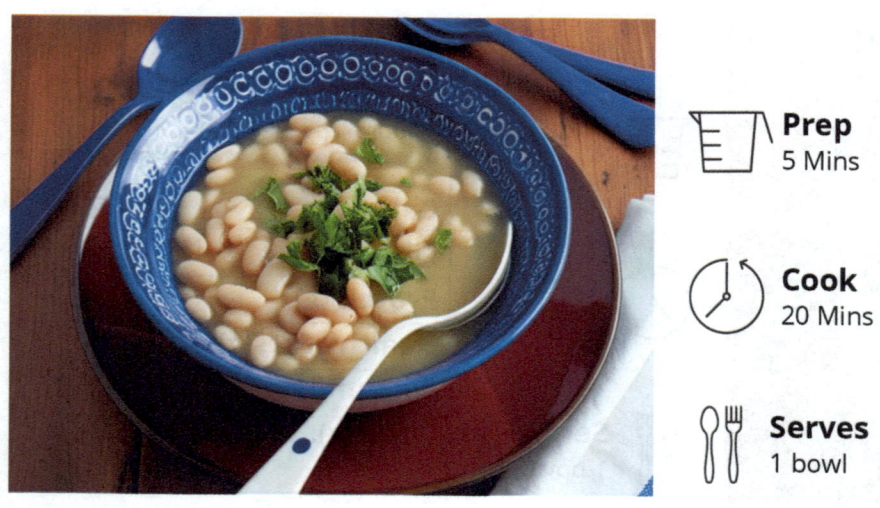

Prep
5 Mins

Cook
20 Mins

Serves
1 bowl

Nutritional Info.
(approx. per serving)

Calories:	250
Fiber(g):	6
Protein(g):	10
Healthy Fats(g):	8
Sodium(mg):	230
Carbs(g):	26

Ingredients

- ½ cup white beans
- ½ cup chopped kale or spinach
- ½ cup diced tomatoes
- 1 cup broth
- 1 garlic clove
- 1 tsp olive oil
- Salt and pepper

Instructions

- Sauté garlic in olive oil.
- Add beans, tomatoes, and broth. Simmer for 10 minutes.
- Add greens and cook until soft.
- Blend partially for creaminess (optional). Serve warm.

Evidence-Based Health Note

White beans offer plant protein and fiber. Greens like kale support digestion and inflammation reduction.

Vegetable Barley Soup

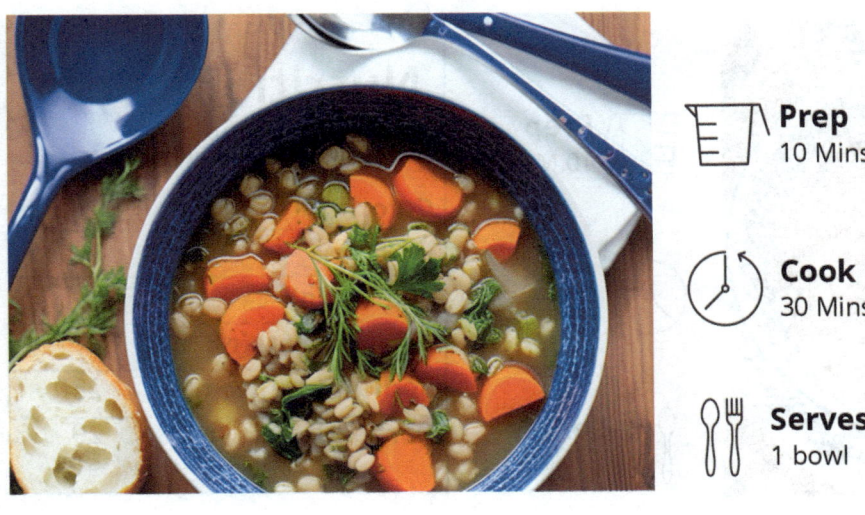

Prep
10 Mins

Cook
30 Mins

Serves
1 bowl

Nutritional Info.
(approx. per serving)

Calories:	220
Fiber(g):	5
Protein(g):	8
Healthy Fats(g):	5
Sodium(mg):	210
Carbs(g):	28

Ingredients

- ¼ cup pearl barley
- ½ cup chopped vegetables (carrots, celery, onion)
- 1 cup vegetable broth
- 1 tsp olive oil
- Salt and pepper

Instructions

- Heat oil in pot, sauté vegetables for 5 minutes.
- Add barley and broth.
- Simmer for 25–30 minutes until barley is tender.
- Season and serve.

Evidence-Based Health Note

Barley provides beta-glucan fiber that improves heart health. Vegetables support immunity and gut function.

Moroccan Lentil Soup

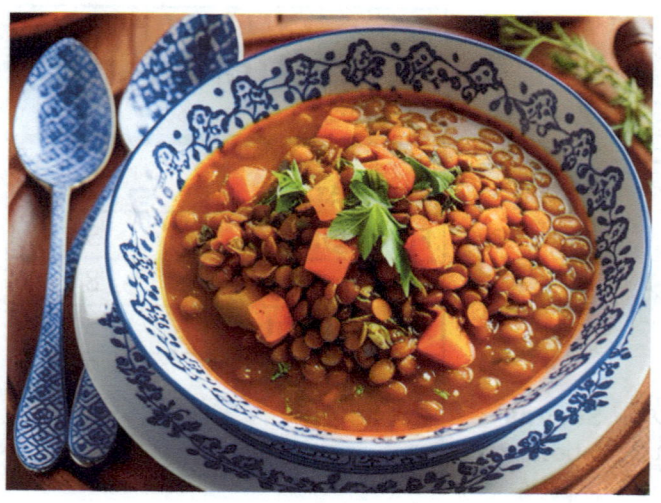

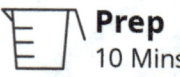 **Prep**
10 Mins

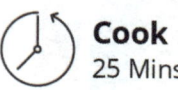 **Cook**
25 Mins

Serves
1 bowl

Nutritional Info.
(approx. per serving)

Calories:	260
Fiber(g):	7
Protein(g):	11
Healthy Fats(g):	6
Sodium(mg):	230
Carbs(g):	29

Ingredients

- ½ cup red lentils
- ¼ cup diced onion
- ½ tsp cumin
- ¼ tsp turmeric
- 1 garlic clove
- 1 cup broth
- 1 tsp olive oil

Instructions

- Heat oil, sauté garlic, onion, and spices.
- Add lentils and broth.
- Simmer for 20–25 minutes until lentils are soft.
- Serve hot with lemon wedge (optional).

Evidence-Based Health Note

Red lentils are rich in folate and fiber. Spices like turmeric have anti-inflammatory benefits.

Hearty Fish Stew with Herbs

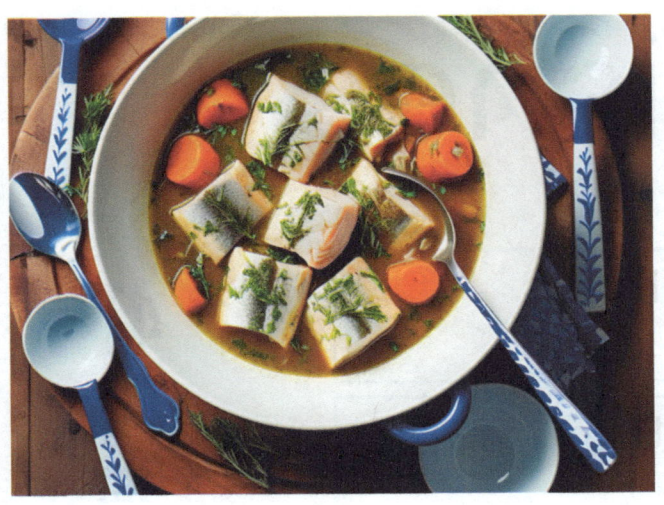

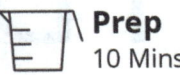
Prep
10 Mins

Cook
20 Mins

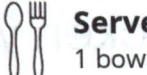
Serves
1 bowl

Nutritional Info.
(approx. per serving)

Calories:	280
Fiber(g):	2
Protein(g):	22
Healthy Fats(g):	9
Sodium(mg):	260
Carbs(g):	14

Ingredients

- 3–4 oz white fish (cod or haddock), cubed
- ½ cup chopped tomato
- ½ cup diced zucchini or bell pepper
- 1 cup broth
- 1 garlic clove
- 1 tsp olive oil
- Fresh parsley or thyme

Instructions

- Sauté garlic and vegetables in olive oil.
- Add tomatoes and broth. Simmer 10 minutes.
- Add fish cubes and cook 8–10 minutes until flaky.
- Garnish with fresh herbs and serve.

Evidence-Based Health Note

White fish provides lean protein and omega-3s that support heart and brain function.

Wholesome Main Dishes

Baked Salmon with Herbs & Olive Tapenade

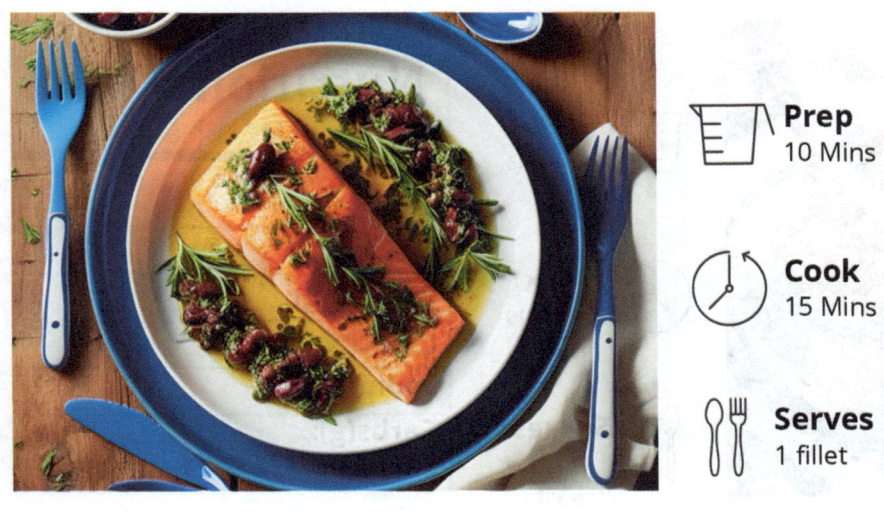

Prep
10 Mins

Cook
15 Mins

Serves
1 fillet

Nutritional Info. (approx. per serving)	
Calories:	320
Fiber(g):	1
Protein(g):	28
Healthy Fats(g):	18
Sodium(mg):	260
Carbs(g):	4

Ingredients

- 1 salmon fillet (4 oz)
- 1 tbsp olive tapenade
- ½ tsp dried thyme or rosemary
- ½ tsp lemon juice
- Salt and pepper

Instructions

- Preheat oven to 375°F (190°C).
- Place salmon on a baking sheet.
- Top with olive tapenade and sprinkle herbs.
- Drizzle with lemon juice.
- Bake for 12–15 minutes or until cooked through.
- Serve warm.

Evidence-Based Health Note

Salmon is a top source of omega-3s, supporting heart and brain health. Olive tapenade adds healthy fats and antioxidants.

Roasted Chicken with Lemon & Rosemary

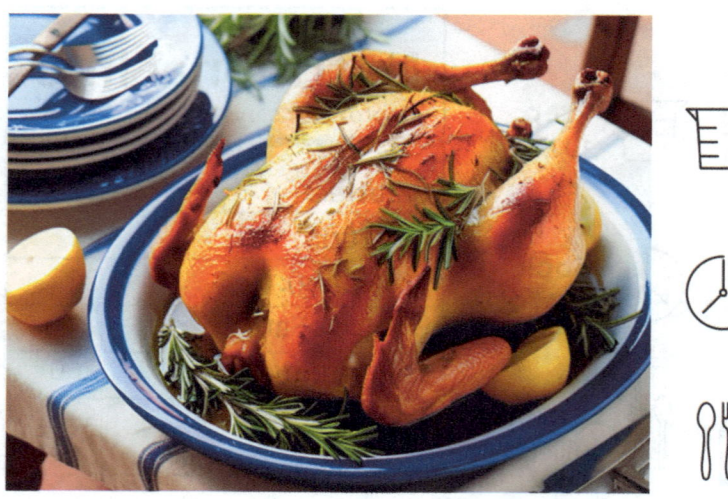

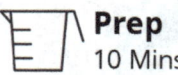 **Prep**
10 Mins

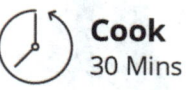 **Cook**
30 Mins

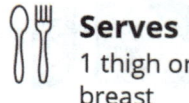 **Serves**
1 thigh or
breast

Nutritional Info.
(approx. per serving)

Calories:	300
Fiber(g):	0
Protein(g):	30
Healthy Fats(g):	14
Sodium(mg):	220
Carbs(g):	2

Ingredients

- 1 chicken thigh or breast (skinless)
- 1 tsp olive oil
- 1 tbsp lemon juice
- ½ tsp dried rosemary
- Salt and pepper

Instructions

- Preheat oven to 400°F (200°C).
- Rub chicken with olive oil, lemon juice, rosemary, salt, and pepper.
- Place in baking dish and roast for 25–30 minutes until juices run clear.
- Let rest 5 minutes before serving.

Evidence-Based Health Note

Chicken provides lean protein for muscle and bone health. Rosemary has anti-inflammatory compounds.

Stuffed Bell Peppers with Quinoa & Veggies

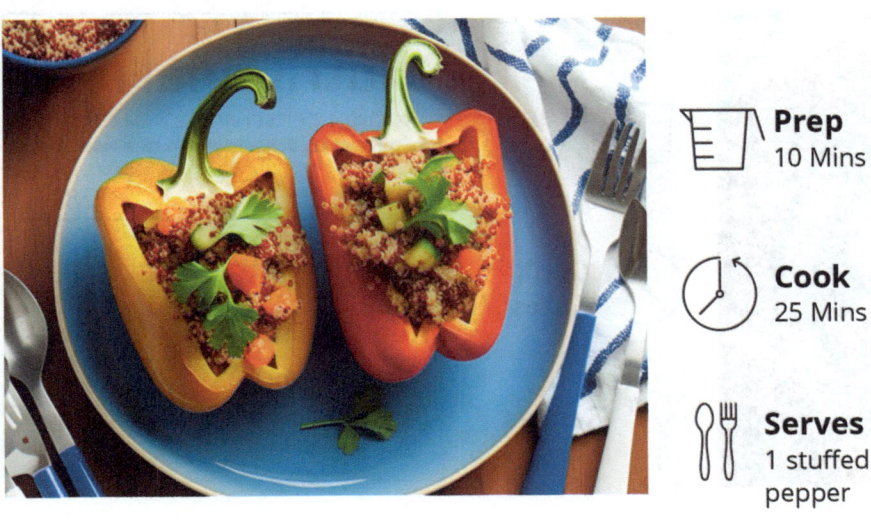

Prep
10 Mins

Cook
25 Mins

Serves
1 stuffed pepper

Nutritional Info.
(approx. per serving)

Calories:	290
Fiber(g):	6
Protein(g):	11
Healthy Fats(g):	10
Sodium(mg):	210
Carbs(g):	30

Ingredients

- 1 bell pepper, halved and seeded
- ½ cup cooked quinoa
- ¼ cup diced tomato
- ¼ cup spinach, chopped
- 1 tsp olive oil
- Salt, pepper, and oregano

Instructions

- Preheat oven to 375°F (190°C).
- Sauté tomato and spinach in olive oil for 3 minutes.
- Mix with quinoa, season, and stuff into pepper halves.
- Bake in a dish with a splash of water, covered, for 25 minutes.
- Serve hot.

Evidence-Based Health Note

Quinoa offers complete plant protein. Bell peppers are rich in vitamin C and antioxidants.

Grilled Shrimp with Garlic & Olive Oil

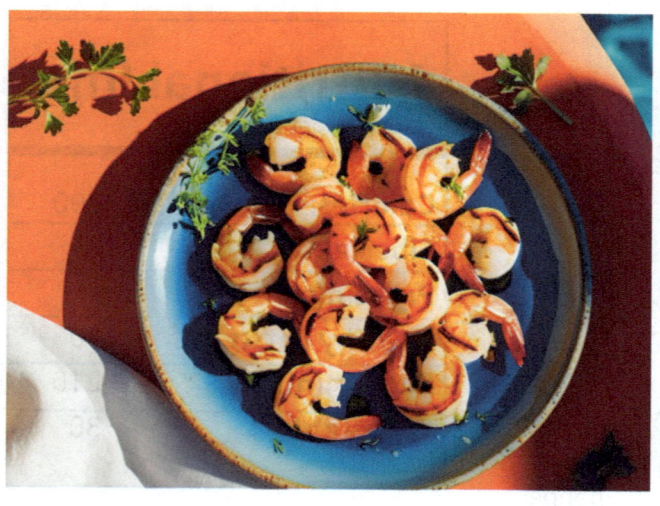

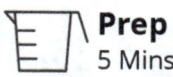 **Prep**
5 Mins

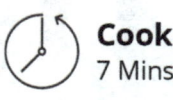 **Cook**
7 Mins

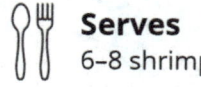 **Serves**
6–8 shrimp

Nutritional Info.
(approx. per serving)

Calories:	280
Fiber(g):	0
Protein(g):	25
Healthy Fats(g):	16
Sodium(mg):	240
Carbs(g):	3

Ingredients

- 6–8 shrimp, peeled and deveined
- 1 tsp olive oil
- 1 garlic clove, minced
- Juice of ¼ lemon
- Salt and pepper

Instructions

- Toss shrimp with olive oil, garlic, lemon juice, salt, and pepper.
- Grill or sauté for 2–3 minutes per side until pink and opaque.
- Serve hot over greens or grains.

Evidence-Based Health Note

Shrimp delivers lean protein and key minerals. Olive oil and garlic promote heart and joint health.

Eggplant Parmesan (Baked)

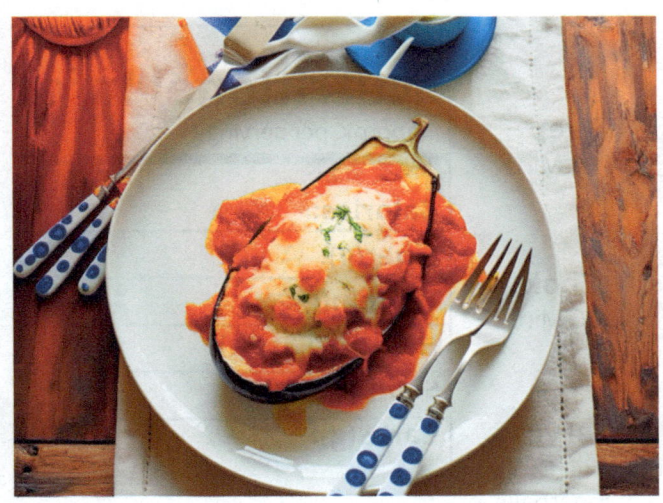

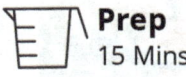 **Prep**
15 Mins

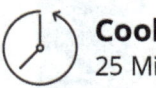 **Cook**
25 Mins

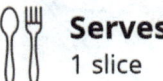 **Serves**
1 slice

Nutritional Info.
(approx. per serving)

Calories:	310
Fiber(g):	5
Protein(g):	14
Healthy Fats(g):	12
Sodium(mg):	320
Carbs(g):	26

Ingredients

- 1 medium eggplant, sliced
- ½ cup marinara sauce
- ¼ cup grated Parmesan cheese
- 1 tsp olive oil
- ½ tsp oregano

Instructions

- Preheat oven to 375°F (190°C).
- Brush eggplant with olive oil and bake for 15 minutes.
- Layer eggplant, marinara, and cheese in a baking dish.
- Top with oregano and bake for another 10 minutes.
- Serve warm.

Evidence-Based Health Note

Eggplant contains antioxidants that may reduce inflammation. Baking reduces saturated fat intake.

Mediterranean Turkey Meatballs

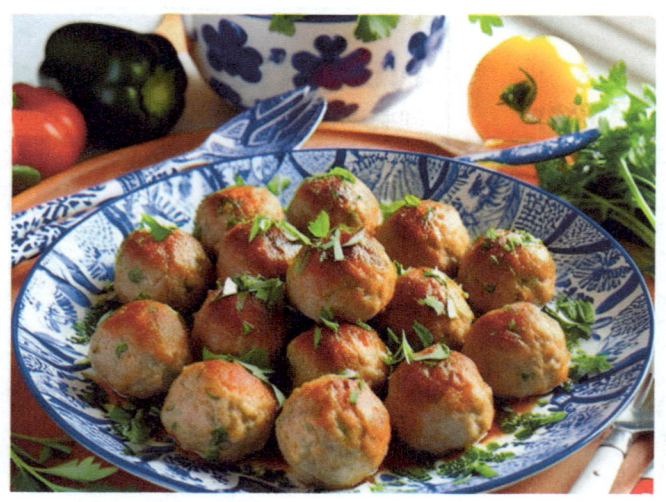

 **Prep**
10 Mins

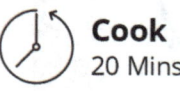 **Cook**
20 Mins

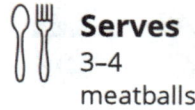 **Serves**
3–4
meatballs

Nutritional Info.
(approx. per serving)

Calories:	270
Fiber(g):	2
Protein(g):	22
Healthy Fats(g):	12
Sodium(mg):	250
Carbs(g):	6

Ingredients

- ½ lb ground turkey
- 1 tbsp chopped parsley
- 1 garlic clove, minced
- 1 egg (or flax egg)
- 1 tbsp breadcrumbs
- 1 tsp olive oil
- Salt and pepper

Instructions

- Preheat oven to 375°F (190°C).
- Mix all ingredients and shape into meatballs.
- Bake for 18–20 minutes until browned and cooked through.
- Serve with tzatziki or tomato sauce.

Evidence-Based Health Note

Turkey is high in protein and low in fat. Herbs and garlic provide anti-inflammatory support.

Baked Falafel with Tahini Sauce

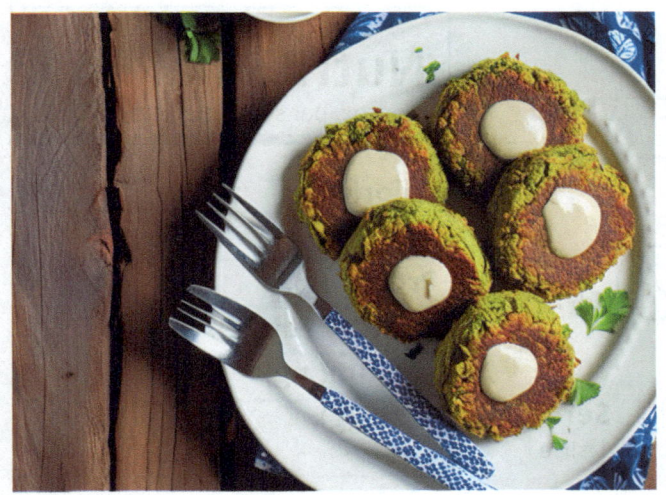

 **Prep**
10 Mins

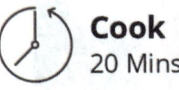 **Cook**
20 Mins

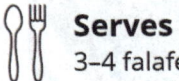 **Serves**
3–4 falafel

Nutritional Info.
(approx. per serving)

Calories:	260
Fiber(g):	5
Protein(g):	10
Healthy Fats(g):	11
Sodium(mg):	230
Carbs(g):	28

Ingredients

- ½ cup canned chickpeas, rinsed
- 1 tbsp chopped onion
- 1 tbsp parsley
- 1 garlic clove
- 1 tsp olive oil
- 1 tbsp tahini
- Pinch of cumin and salt

Instructions

- Preheat oven to 375°F (190°C).
- Blend chickpeas, onion, parsley, garlic, and spices until chunky.
- Form into balls, brush with oil, and bake for 20 minutes.
- Drizzle with tahini to serve.

Evidence-Based Health Note

Chickpeas support heart and digestive health. Tahini adds calcium and healthy fats.

Vegetable Moussaka

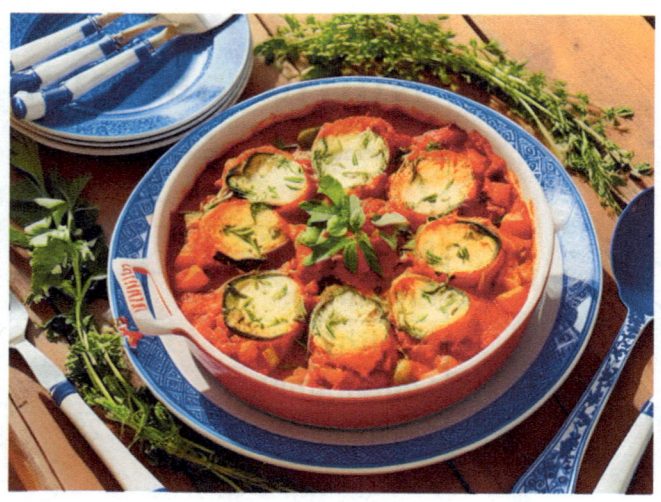

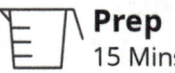
Prep
15 Mins

Cook
35 Mins

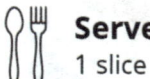
Serves
1 slice

Nutritional Info.
(approx. per serving)

Calories:	310
Fiber(g):	4
Protein(g):	13
Healthy Fats(g):	15
Sodium(mg):	280
Carbs(g):	20

Ingredients

- ½ cup sliced eggplant
- ¼ cup chopped zucchini
- ¼ cup crushed tomatoes
- 2 tbsp feta or ricotta
- 1 tsp olive oil
- Pinch of cinnamon

Instructions

- Sauté eggplant and zucchini in olive oil until soft.
- Layer with tomatoes, feta, and cinnamon in a small dish.
- Bake at 375°F (190°C) for 30–35 minutes.
- Cool slightly before serving.

Evidence-Based Health Note

Vegetables provide fiber and antioxidants. Cheese offers calcium to support bone health.

Tuna-Stuffed Tomatoes

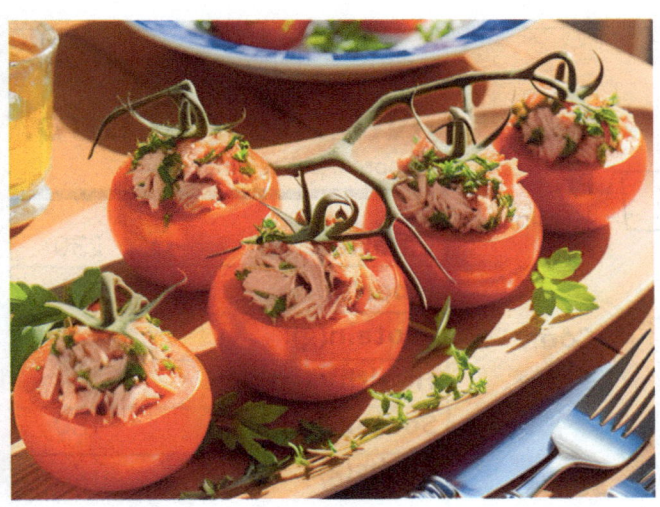

 **Prep**
10 Mins

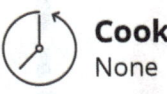 **Cook**
None

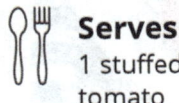 **Serves**
1 stuffed
tomato

Nutritional Info.
(approx. per serving)

Calories:	240
Fiber(g):	3
Protein(g):	18
Healthy Fats(g):	10
Sodium(mg):	200
Carbs(g):	8

Ingredients

- 1 large tomato
- ¼ cup canned tuna
- 1 tsp olive oil
- ½ tbsp chopped celery
- Lemon juice, salt, pepper

Instructions

- Cut top off tomato and scoop out seeds.
- Mix tuna with oil, celery, lemon juice, and seasoning.
- Stuff tomato with mixture.
- Chill or serve immediately.

Evidence-Based Health Note

Tuna delivers omega-3s for brain and heart support. Tomatoes are rich in lycopene.

Zucchini Noodles with Pesto & Cherry Tomatoes

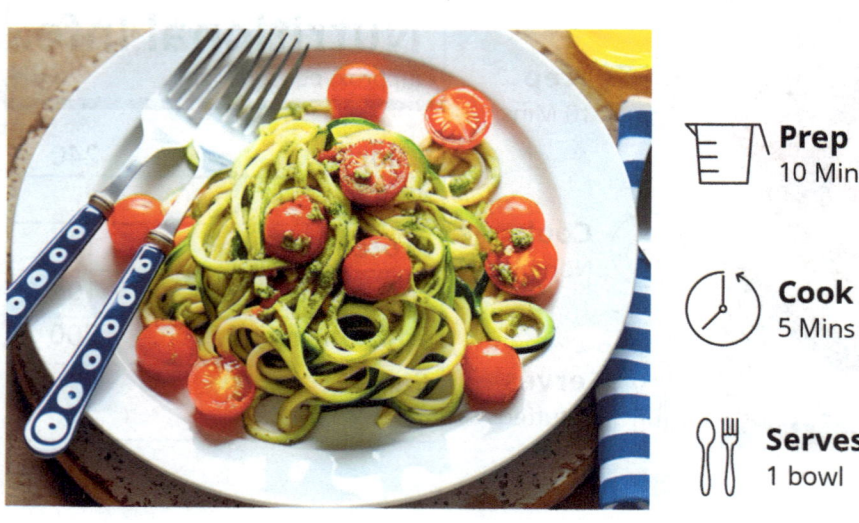

Prep
10 Mins

Cook
5 Mins

Serves
1 bowl

Nutritional Info.	
(approx. per serving)	
Calories:	230
Fiber(g):	3
Protein(g):	9
Healthy Fats(g):	12
Sodium(mg):	180
Carbs(g):	12

Ingredients

- 1 medium zucchini, spiralized
- ¼ cup cherry tomatoes, halved
- 1 tbsp pesto
- 1 tsp olive oil

Instructions

- Sauté zucchini noodles in olive oil for 2–3 minutes.
- Add cherry tomatoes and cook 1–2 minutes.
- Toss with pesto and serve warm.

Evidence-Based Health Note

Zucchini is low-carb and hydrating. Pesto and tomatoes provide heart-healthy fats and antioxidants.

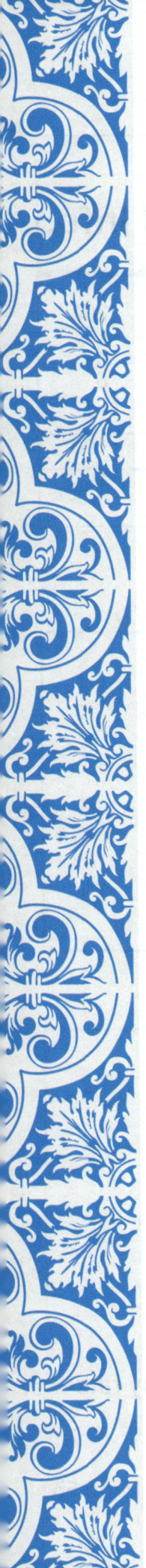

Simple Sides & Veggie Mains

Roasted Cauliflower with Tahini

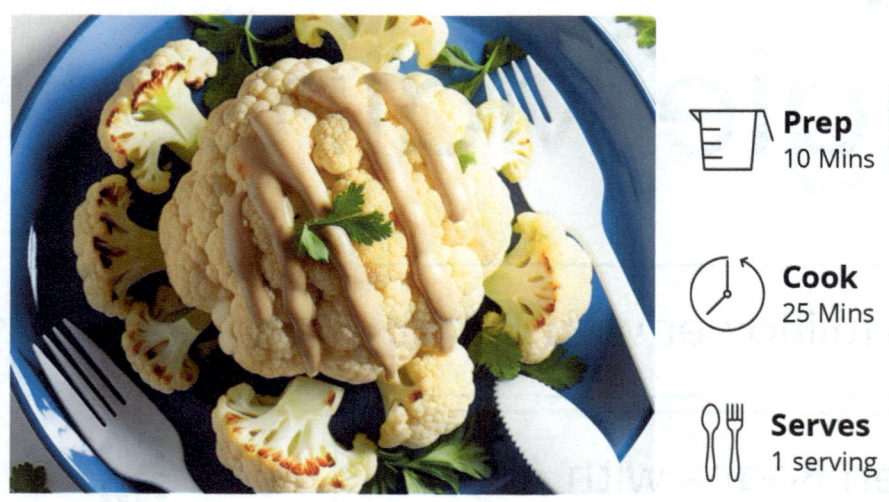

Prep
10 Mins

Cook
25 Mins

Serves
1 serving

Nutritional Info.	
(approx. per serving)	
Calories:	200
Fiber(g):	5
Protein(g):	6
Healthy Fats(g):	12
Sodium(mg):	180
Carbs(g):	16

Ingredients

- 1 cup cauliflower florets
- 1 tsp olive oil
- 1 tbsp tahini
- ½ tbsp lemon juice
- Pinch of cumin
- Salt and pepper

Instructions

- Preheat oven to 400°F (200°C).
- Toss cauliflower with olive oil, salt, and cumin.
- Roast for 25 minutes until golden.
- Mix tahini, lemon juice, and a splash of water to make sauce.
- Drizzle sauce over roasted cauliflower. Serve warm.

Evidence-Based Health Note

Cauliflower provides fiber and antioxidants. Tahini offers calcium and healthy fats for joint and bone support.

Garlic Green Beans with Almonds

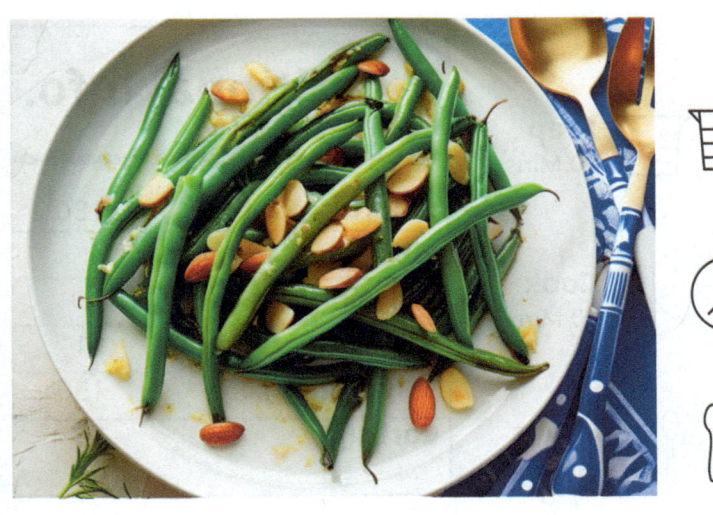

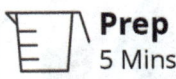 **Prep**
5 Mins

 **Cook**
10 Mins

 **Serves**
1 serving

Nutritional Info.
(approx. per serving)

Calories:	170
Fiber(g):	4
Protein(g):	5
Healthy Fats(g):	9
Sodium(mg):	160
Carbs(g):	12

Ingredients

- 1 cup green beans, trimmed
- 1 garlic clove, minced
- 1 tsp olive oil
- 1 tbsp sliced almonds
- Salt to taste

Instructions

- Steam green beans for 5 minutes.
- Sauté garlic in olive oil, then add beans.
- Cook for 2–3 minutes.
- Sprinkle with almonds before serving.

Evidence-Based Health Note

Green beans are rich in vitamin K and fiber. Almonds add healthy fats and magnesium for heart support.

Grilled Eggplant with Olive Oil & Herbs

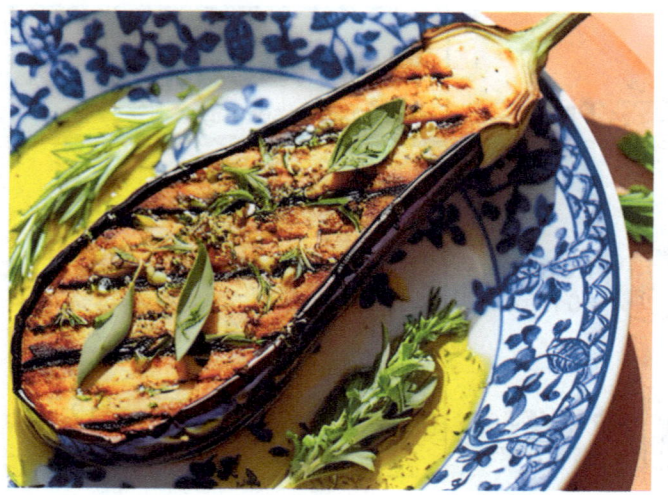

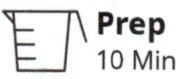 **Prep**
10 Mins

 **Cook**
10 Mins

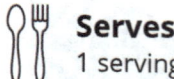 **Serves**
1 serving

Nutritional Info.
(approx. per serving)

Calories:	180
Fiber(g):	5
Protein(g):	3
Healthy Fats(g):	11
Sodium(mg):	150
Carbs(g):	15

Ingredients

- ½ medium eggplant, sliced
- 1 tsp olive oil
- ½ tsp mixed herbs (oregano, thyme)
- Salt and pepper

Instructions

- Brush eggplant slices with oil and season.
- Grill 3–4 minutes per side.
- Sprinkle herbs and serve.

Evidence-Based Health Note

Eggplant delivers antioxidants like nasunin. Olive oil supports heart and joint health.

Steamed Broccoli with Lemon & Olive Oil

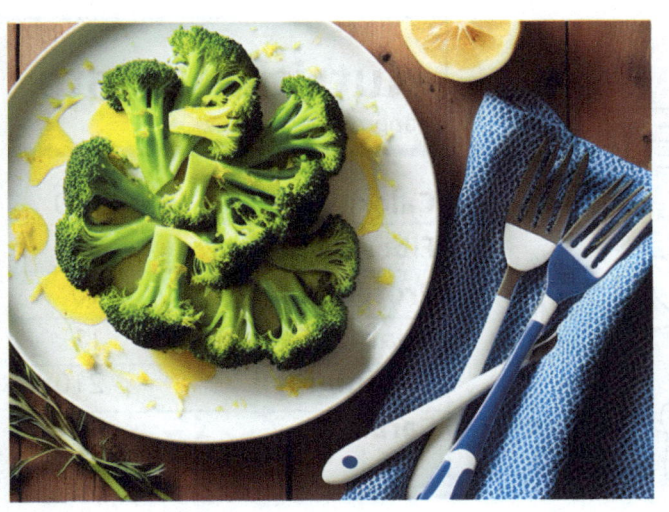

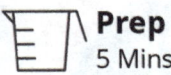 **Prep**
5 Mins

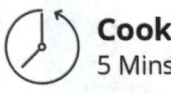 **Cook**
5 Mins

 **Serves**
1 serving

Nutritional Info.
(approx. per serving)

Calories:	140
Fiber(g):	5
Protein(g):	4
Healthy Fats(g):	8
Sodium(mg):	120
Carbs(g):	10

Ingredients

- 1 cup broccoli florets
- 1 tsp olive oil
- ½ tbsp lemon juice
- Pinch of salt

Instructions

- Steam broccoli for 4–5 minutes until tender.
- Drizzle with olive oil and lemon juice.
- Sprinkle salt and serve warm.

Evidence-Based Health Note

Broccoli is packed with vitamin C and calcium. Lemon enhances iron absorption.

Chickpea Patties with Yogurt Sauce

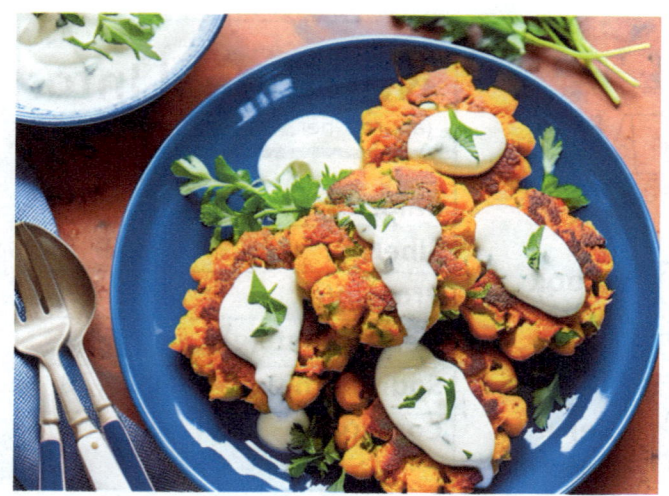

Prep
10 Mins

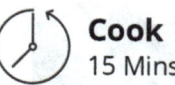
Cook
15 Mins

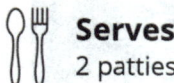
Serves
2 patties

Nutritional Info.
(approx. per serving)

Calories:	250
Fiber(g):	6
Protein(g):	10
Healthy Fats(g):	11
Sodium(mg):	210
Carbs(g):	24

Ingredients

- ½ cup canned chickpeas, mashed
- 1 tbsp chopped onion
- 1 tbsp parsley
- 1 tbsp whole wheat flour
- 1 tsp olive oil
- 2 tbsp plain yogurt + ½ tsp lemon juice for sauce

Instructions

- Mix mashed chickpeas, onion, parsley, and flour.
- Form into patties and sauté in olive oil until golden.
- Combine yogurt and lemon for sauce.
- Serve with patties.

Evidence-Based Health Note

Chickpeas support heart and digestive health. Yogurt adds calcium and probiotics.

Sweet Potato Wedges with Paprika

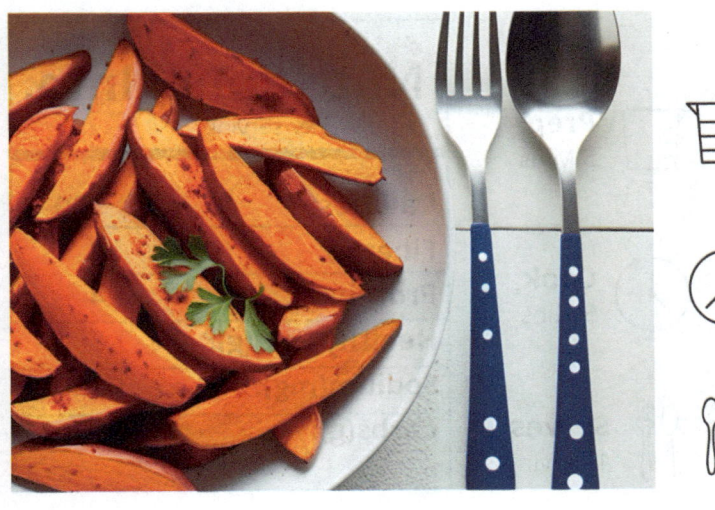

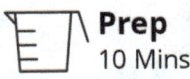

Prep
10 Mins

Cook
25 Mins

Serves
1 serving

Nutritional Info.
(approx. per serving)

Calories:	220
Fiber(g):	4
Protein(g):	3
Healthy Fats(g):	10
Sodium(mg):	140
Carbs(g):	28

Ingredients

- 1 small sweet potato, cut into wedges
- 1 tsp olive oil
- ½ tsp paprika
- Salt to taste

Instructions

- Preheat oven to 400°F (200°C).
- Toss wedges with oil, paprika, and salt.
- Bake for 25 minutes, flipping halfway through.
- Serve warm.

Evidence-Based Health Note

Sweet potatoes are high in beta-carotene and fiber. Paprika adds anti-inflammatory benefits.

Spinach Sautéed with Garlic

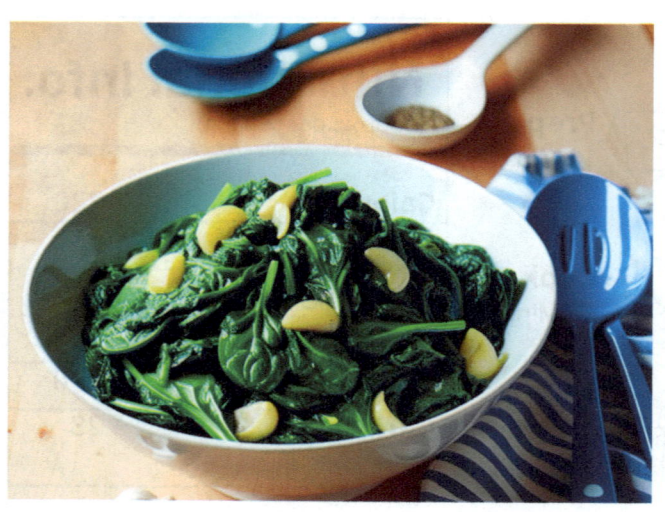

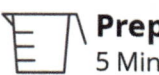

Prep
5 Mins

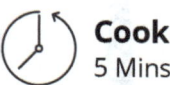

Cook
5 Mins

Serves
1 serving

Nutritional Info.
(approx. per serving)

Calories:	130
Fiber(g):	3
Protein(g):	4
Healthy Fats(g):	8
Sodium(mg):	150
Carbs(g):	7

Ingredients

- 1 cup fresh spinach
- 1 garlic clove, minced
- 1 tsp olive oil
- Pinch of salt

Instructions

- Heat oil and sauté garlic until fragrant.
- Add spinach and cook until wilted (about 2 minutes).
- Season and serve.

Evidence-Based Health Note

Spinach offers iron and folate for brain and blood health. Garlic has heart-protective properties.

Zucchini Fritters with Dill Yogurt

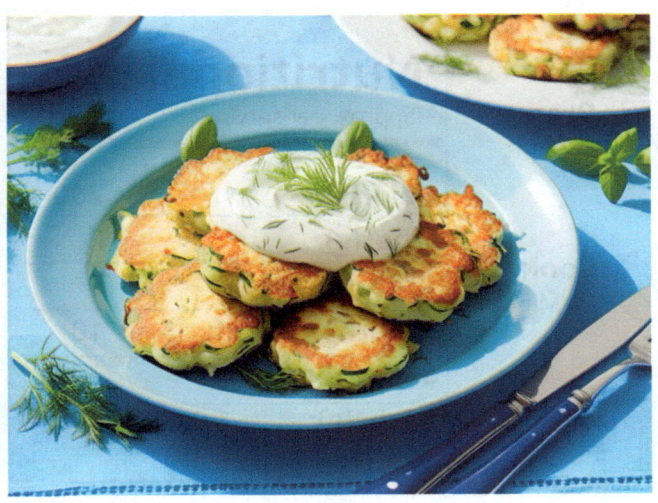

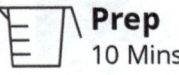
Prep
10 Mins

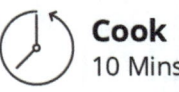
Cook
10 Mins

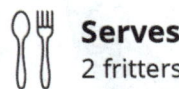
Serves
2 fritters

Nutritional Info.
(approx. per serving)

Calories:	240
Fiber(g):	3
Protein(g):	8
Healthy Fats(g):	11
Sodium(mg):	180
Carbs(g):	20

Ingredients

- ½ cup grated zucchini
- 1 tbsp chopped onion
- 1 tbsp whole wheat flour
- 1 egg or flax egg
- 1 tsp olive oil
- 2 tbsp plain yogurt + chopped dill

Instructions

- Squeeze moisture from grated zucchini.
- Mix with onion, flour, and egg.
- Form small fritters and cook in olive oil 3–4 min/side.
- Serve with dill yogurt.

Evidence-Based Health Note

Zucchini supports hydration and digestion. Yogurt adds calcium and gut-friendly probiotics.

Stuffed Mushrooms with Herbs & Cheese

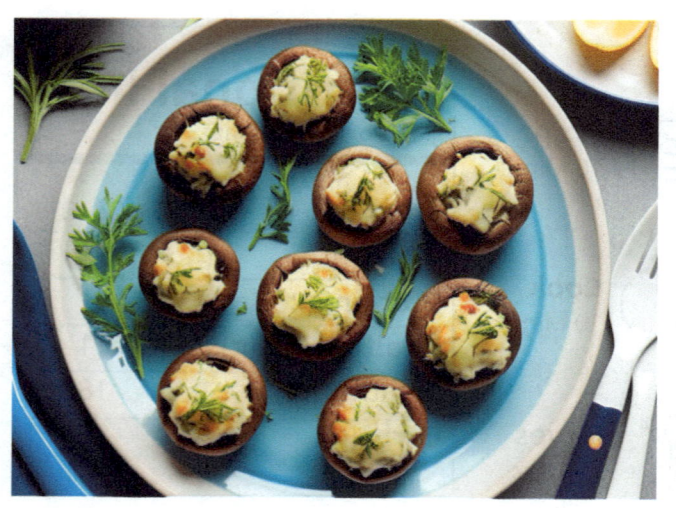

 **Prep**
10 Mins

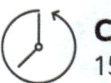 **Cook**
15 Mins

 Serves
3 stuffed mushrooms

Nutritional Info.
(approx. per serving)

Calories:	200
Fiber(g):	2
Protein(g):	9
Healthy Fats(g):	10
Sodium(mg):	200
Carbs(g):	10

Ingredients

- 3 large mushrooms, stems removed
- 1 tbsp feta or ricotta cheese
- ½ tbsp chopped parsley
- ½ tsp olive oil
- Salt and pepper

Instructions

- Mix cheese, parsley, salt, and pepper.
- Fill mushroom caps with mixture.
- Drizzle with olive oil and bake at 375°F (190°C) for 15 minutes.

Evidence-Based Health Note

Mushrooms are anti-inflammatory and immune-supportive. Cheese adds protein and calcium.

Couscous with Roasted Vegetables

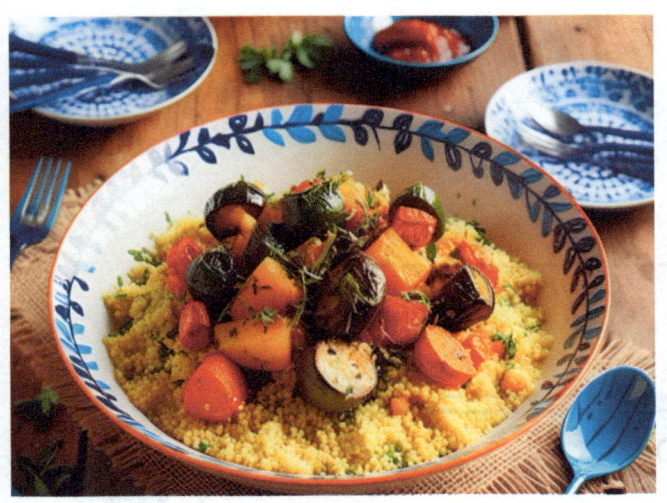

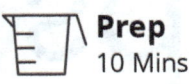

Prep
10 Mins

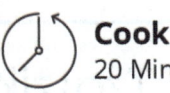

Cook
20 Mins

Serves
1 bowl

Nutritional Info.
(approx. per serving)

Calories:	270
Fiber(g):	5
Protein(g):	7
Healthy Fats(g):	10
Sodium(mg):	190
Carbs(g):	35

Ingredients

- ½ cup cooked couscous
- ½ cup diced roasted vegetables (zucchini, bell pepper, onion)
- 1 tsp olive oil
- ½ tsp lemon juice
- Pinch of cumin

Instructions

- Roast vegetables with olive oil at 400°F (200°C) for 20 minutes.
- Mix with cooked couscous.
- Add lemon juice and cumin. Serve warm or cold.

Evidence-Based Health Note

Couscous provides energy and selenium. Roasted vegetables deliver fiber and antioxidants.

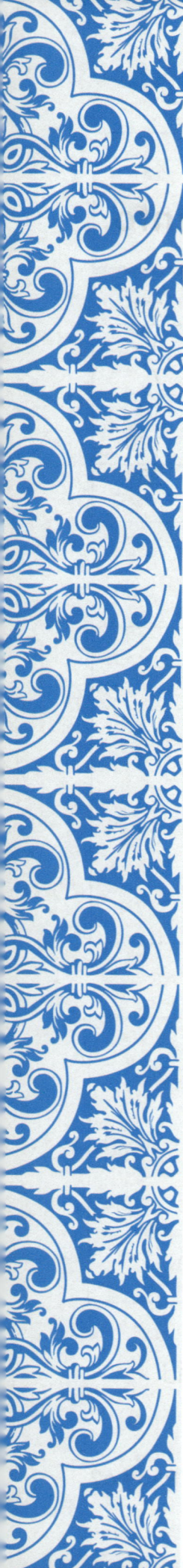

Tasty Snacks & Dips

Homemade Tzatziki

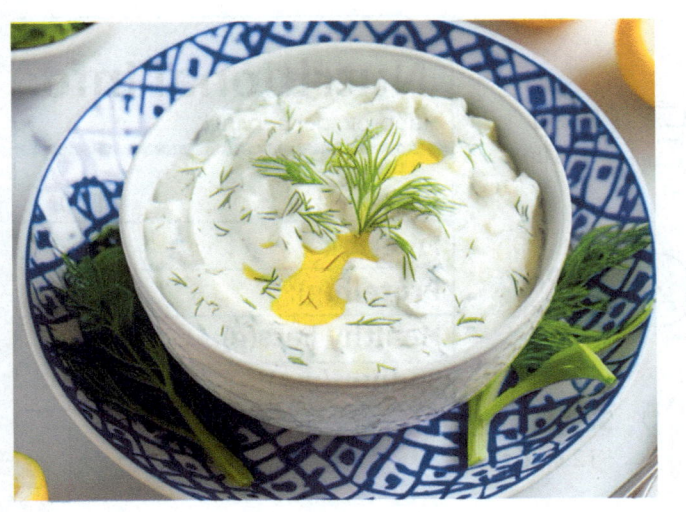

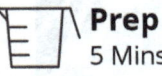 **Prep**
5 Mins

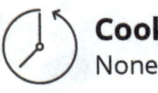 **Cook**
None

 **Serves**
~2 tbsp

Nutritional Info.
(approx. per serving)

Calories:	90
Fiber(g):	0
Protein(g):	4
Healthy Fats(g):	6
Sodium(mg):	100
Carbs(g):	3

Ingredients

- ½ cup plain Greek yogurt
- ¼ cup grated cucumber (squeezed dry)
- 1 tsp lemon juice
- ½ clove garlic, minced
- ½ tsp olive oil
- Pinch of salt

Instructions

- In a bowl, combine yogurt, cucumber, lemon juice, garlic, olive oil, and salt.
- Mix until smooth and creamy.
- Chill briefly or serve immediately as a dip.

Evidence-Based Health Note

Greek yogurt provides protein and probiotics. Cucumber adds hydration and digestive support.

Baked Zucchini Chips with Oregano

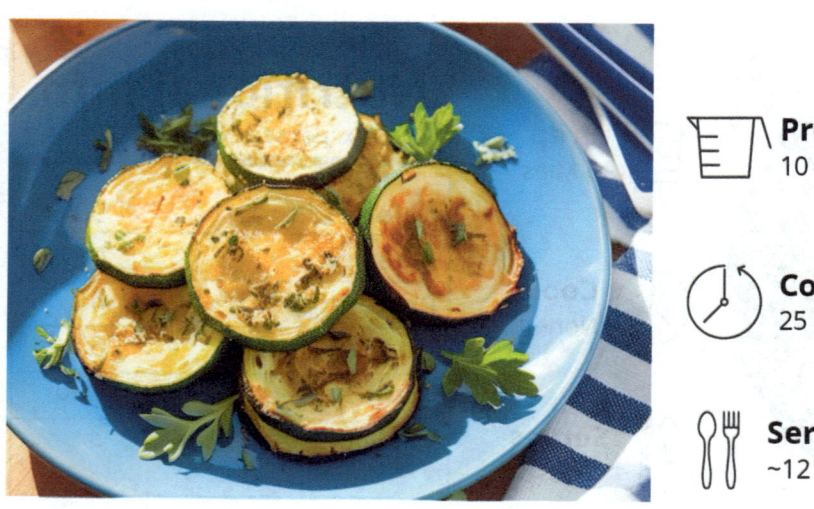

Prep
10 Mins

Cook
25 Mins

Serves
~12 chips

Nutritional Info.
(approx. per serving)

Calories:	110
Fiber(g):	2
Protein(g):	3
Healthy Fats(g):	7
Sodium(mg):	150
Carbs(g):	8

Ingredients

- 1 small zucchini, thinly sliced
- 1 tsp olive oil
- ½ tsp dried oregano
- Pinch of salt

Instructions

- Preheat oven to 400°F (200°C).
- Toss zucchini slices with olive oil, oregano, and salt.
- Arrange in a single layer on a baking sheet.
- Bake for 20–25 minutes until crisp, flipping once.

Evidence-Based Health Note

Zucchini supports hydration and digestion. Oregano offers antimicrobial and anti-inflammatory benefits.

Roasted Chickpeas

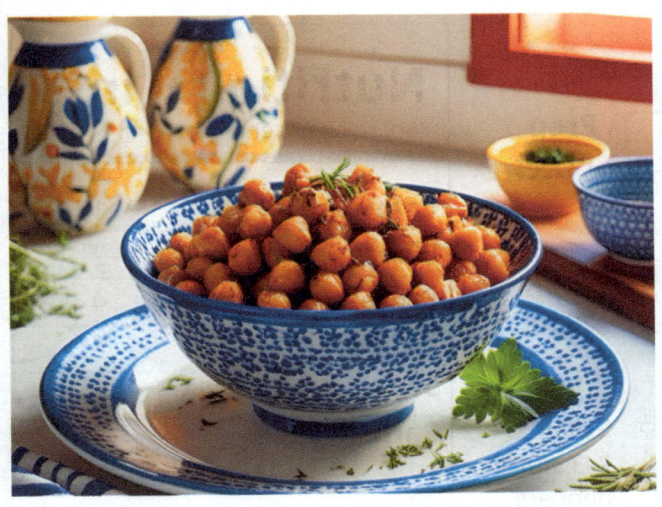

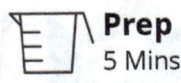

Prep
5 Mins

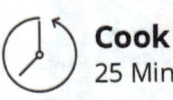

Cook
25 Mins

Serves
¼ cup

Nutritional Info.
(approx. per serving)

Calories:	140
Fiber(g):	4
Protein(g):	6
Healthy Fats(g):	5
Sodium(mg):	180
Carbs(g):	16

Ingredients

- ½ cup canned chickpeas, rinsed and dried
- 1 tsp olive oil
- ½ tsp paprika or cumin
- Pinch of salt

Instructions

- Preheat oven to 400°F (200°C).
- Toss chickpeas with oil, spice, and salt.
- Spread on a baking sheet and roast for 25 minutes, shaking halfway.
- Let cool before serving.

Evidence-Based Health Note

Chickpeas are high in fiber and plant protein, supporting heart and digestive health.

Stuffed Mini Bell Peppers with Feta

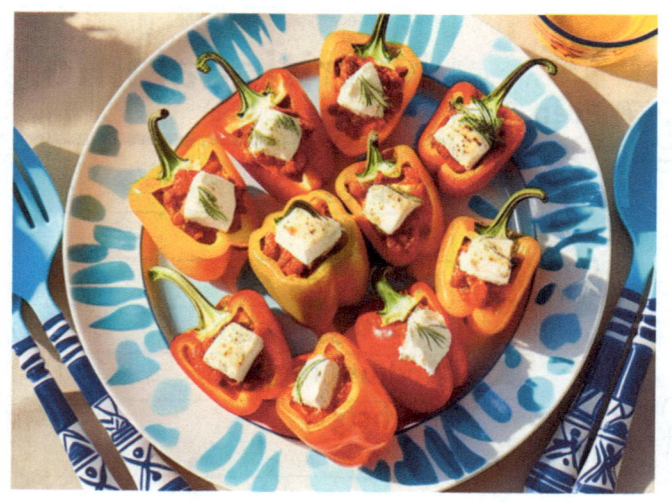

Prep
10 Mins

Cook
None

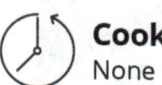

Serves
2–3 stuffed peppers

Nutritional Info.
(approx. per serving)

Calories:	120
Fiber(g):	2
Protein(g):	4
Healthy Fats(g):	7
Sodium(mg):	160
Carbs(g):	9

Ingredients

- 3 mini bell peppers, halved and seeded
- 2 tbsp crumbled feta cheese
- 1 tsp olive oil
- Pinch of oregano

Instructions

- Stuff each pepper half with a bit of feta.
- Drizzle with olive oil and sprinkle oregano.
- Serve fresh and chilled.

Evidence-Based Health Note

Bell peppers are rich in vitamin C. Feta provides calcium for bone strength.

Olive Tapenade with Whole-Grain Crackers

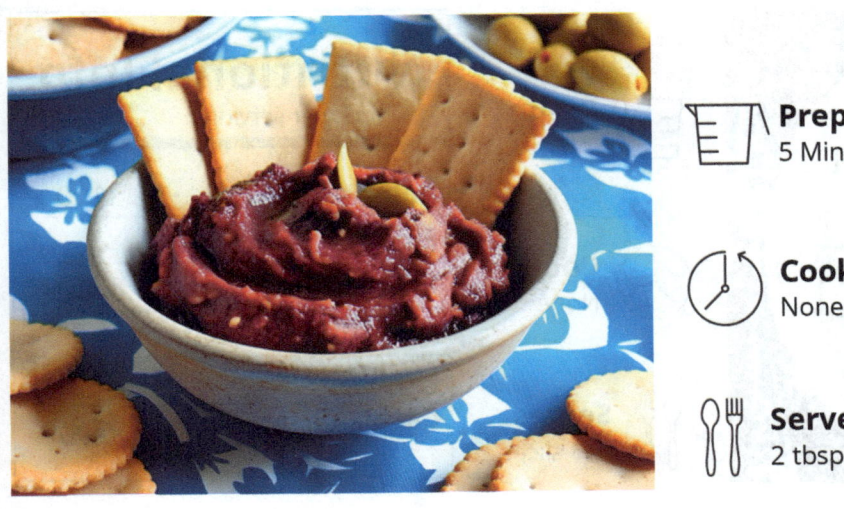
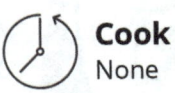

Prep
5 Mins

Cook
None

Serves
2 tbsp

Nutritional Info.
(approx. per serving)

Calories:	130
Fiber(g):	2
Protein(g):	2
Healthy Fats(g):	9
Sodium(mg):	240
Carbs(g):	10

Ingredients

- ¼ cup pitted olives (Kalamata or black)
- ½ tbsp olive oil
- ½ tsp lemon juice
- ¼ clove garlic
- Whole-grain crackers (for serving)

Instructions

- Pulse olives, olive oil, lemon juice, and garlic in a food processor until chunky.
- Serve with crackers or veggie sticks.

Evidence-Based Health Note

Olives contain heart-healthy fats and antioxidants. Whole grains support digestion.

Cucumber Slices with Hummus

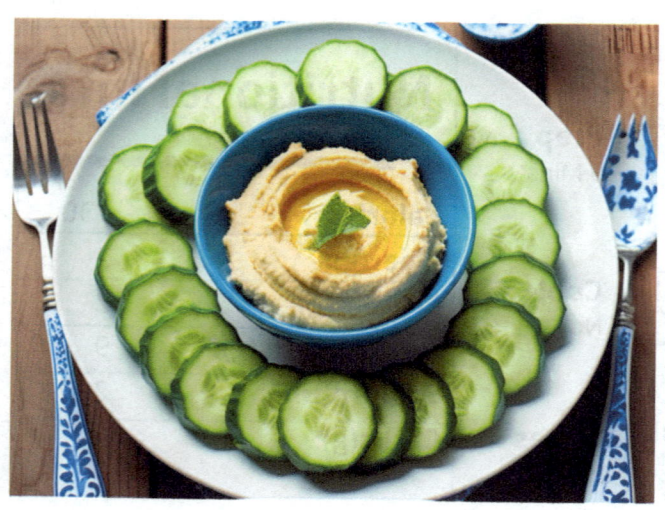

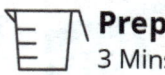
Prep
3 Mins

Cook
None

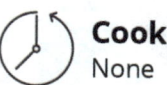
Serves
6–8 slices

Nutritional Info.
(approx. per serving)

Calories:	100
Fiber(g):	2
Protein(g):	3
Healthy Fats(g):	5
Sodium(mg):	120
Carbs(g):	9

Ingredients

- ½ cucumber, sliced
- 2 tbsp hummus

Instructions

- Slice cucumber into rounds.
- Spoon a small dollop of hummus on each slice or serve on the side as a dip.

Evidence-Based Health Note

Cucumbers aid hydration. Hummus offers fiber, protein, and heart-healthy fats.

Sun-Dried Tomato & Basil Spread

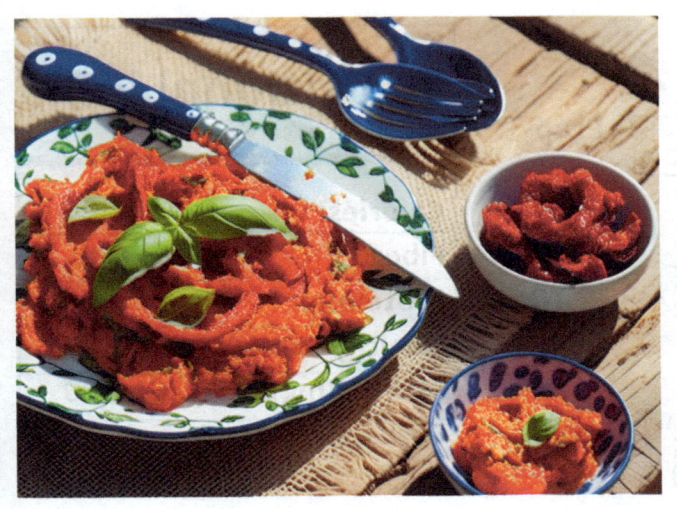

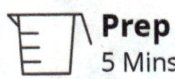
Prep
5 Mins

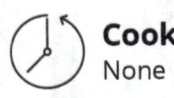
Cook
None

Serves
2 tbsp

Nutritional Info.
(approx. per serving)

Calories:	110
Fiber(g):	1
Protein(g):	2
Healthy Fats(g):	8
Sodium(mg):	170
Carbs(g):	6

Ingredients

- 3 sun-dried tomatoes (in oil), chopped
- ½ tbsp olive oil
- 1 tbsp plain Greek yogurt or ricotta
- ½ tsp chopped fresh basil

Instructions

- Blend tomatoes, olive oil, yogurt/ricotta, and basil until smooth.
- Use as a dip, sandwich spread, or topping for toast.

Evidence-Based Health Note

Sun-dried tomatoes are rich in lycopene. Basil adds antioxidants and anti-inflammatory compounds.

Avocado Dip with Lemon & Garlic

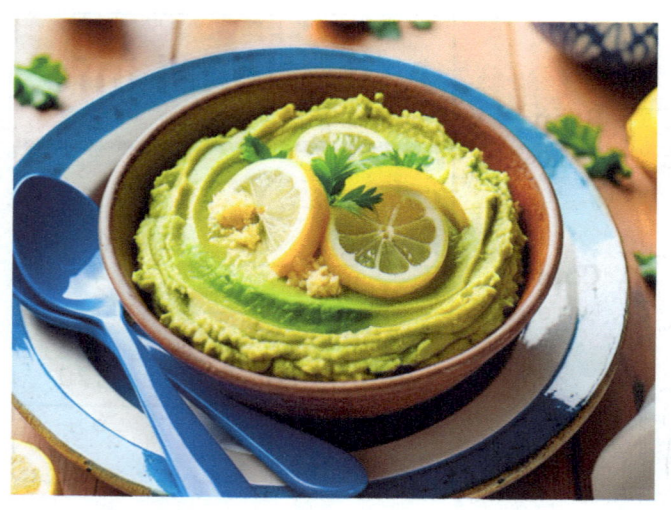

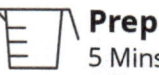 **Prep**
5 Mins

Cook
None

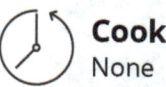 **Serves**
~2–3 tbsp

Nutritional Info.
(approx. per serving)

Calories:	130
Fiber(g):	3
Protein(g):	2
Healthy Fats(g):	10
Sodium(mg):	100
Carbs(g):	7

Ingredients

- ½ ripe avocado
- 1 tsp lemon juice
- 1 small garlic clove, minced (or ⅛ tsp garlic powder)
- 1 tsp olive oil
- Pinch of salt and black pepper

Instructions

- In a small bowl, mash the avocado with a fork until smooth.
- Add lemon juice, garlic, olive oil, salt, and pepper.
- Mix well until creamy.
- Serve immediately with raw veggies or whole-grain crackers.

Evidence-Based Health Note

Avocado delivers monounsaturated fats for heart health. Garlic supports immune and cardiovascular function.

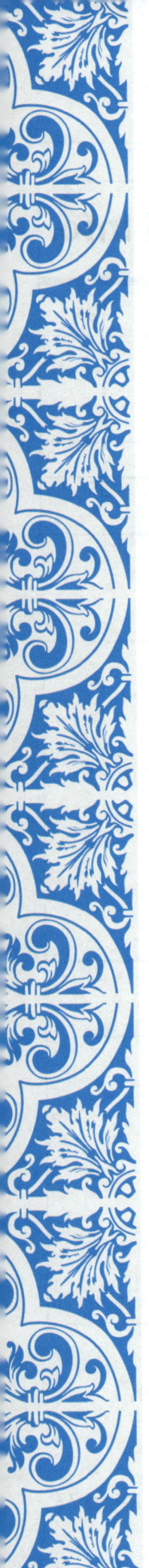

Light & Healthy Desserts

Baked Apples with Cinnamon

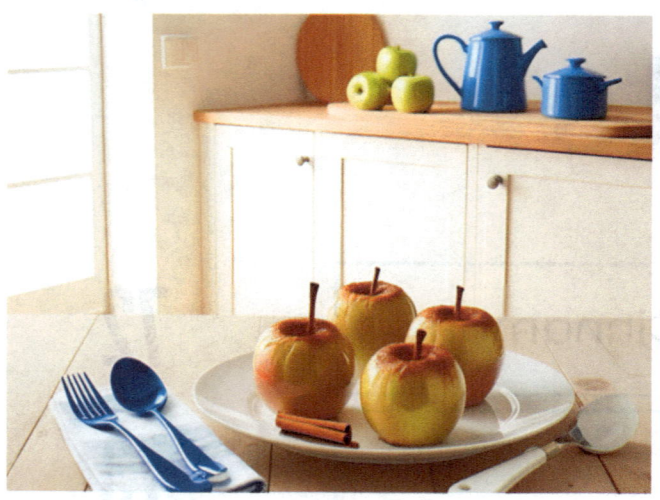

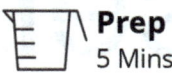 **Prep**
5 Mins

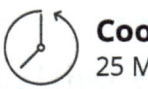 **Cook**
25 Mins

 **Serves**
1 small
apple

Nutritional Info.	
(approx. per serving)	
Calories:	160
Fiber(g):	4
Protein(g):	1
Healthy Fats(g):	2
Sodium(mg):	0
Carbs(g):	35

Ingredients

- 1 small apple, cored
- ½ tsp cinnamon
- ½ tsp honey (optional)
- 1 tsp chopped walnuts (optional)

Instructions

- Preheat oven to 375°F (190°C).
- Place apple in a small baking dish.
- Sprinkle cinnamon into the center and drizzle honey, if using.
- Add walnuts if desired.
- Bake for 25 minutes or until soft.
- Let cool slightly before serving.

Evidence-Based Health Note

Apples provide fiber and polyphenols that support digestion and heart health.
Cinnamon has anti-inflammatory properties.

Honey Yogurt with Toasted Pistachios

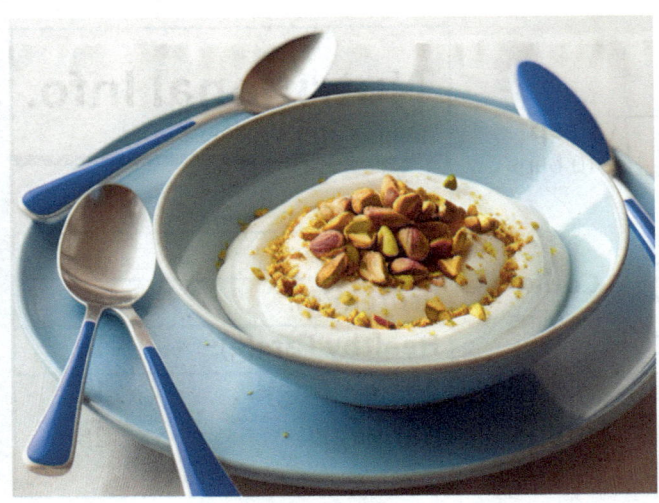

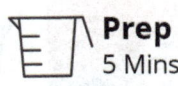
Prep
5 Mins

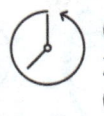
Cook
2 minutes
(to toast
nuts)

Serves
½ cup

Nutritional Info.
(approx. per serving)

Calories:	180
Fiber(g):	1
Protein(g):	7
Healthy Fats(g):	7
Sodium(mg):	40
Carbs(g):	20

Ingredients

- ½ cup plain Greek yogurt
- 1 tsp honey
- 1 tbsp chopped pistachios

Instructions

- Toast pistachios in a dry pan over low heat for 2–3 minutes.
- Spoon yogurt into a bowl.
- Drizzle honey on top.
- Sprinkle with warm pistachios and serve.

Evidence-Based Health Note

Greek yogurt offers protein and calcium. Pistachios contain antioxidants and healthy fats.

Olive Oil Orange Cake (Mini Slice)

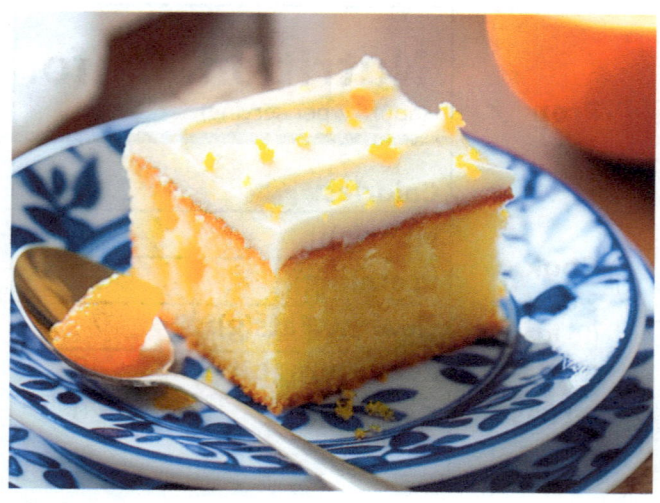

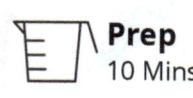 **Prep**
10 Mins

Cook
30 Mins

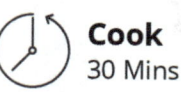 **Serves**
1 mini slice

Nutritional Info.
(approx. per serving)

Calories:	210
Fiber(g):	1
Protein(g):	3
Healthy Fats(g):	10
Sodium(mg):	120
Carbs(g):	28

Ingredients

- ½ cup flour
- ¼ tsp baking powder
- 2 tbsp olive oil
- 2 tbsp orange juice
- 1 tbsp honey
- 1 egg (or flax egg)
- Zest of ½ orange

Instructions

- Preheat oven to 350°F (175°C).
- Mix dry ingredients in one bowl; wet ingredients in another.
- Combine and stir until smooth.
- Pour into greased mini loaf pan or muffin tin.
- Bake 25–30 minutes. Cool before slicing.

Evidence-Based Health Note

Olive oil delivers heart-healthy fats. Oranges are rich in vitamin C and flavonoids.

Frozen Banana Bites with Dark Chocolate

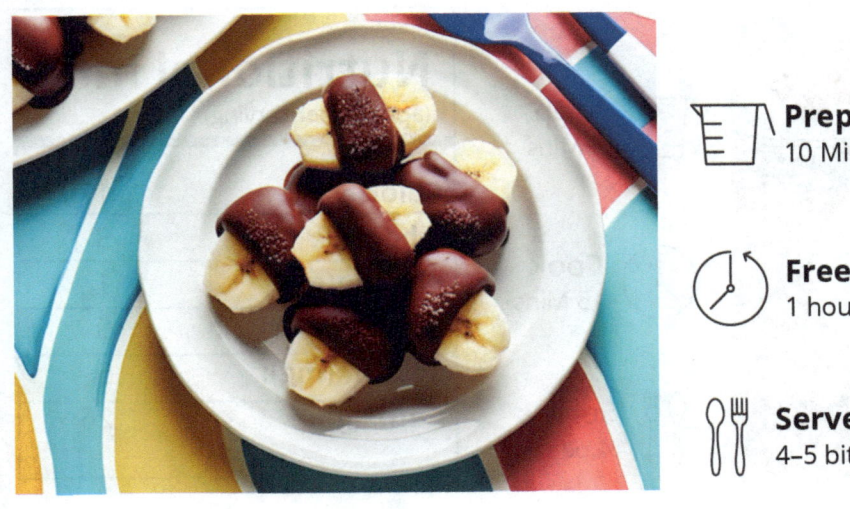

Prep
10 Mins

Freeze
1 hour

Serves
4–5 bites

Nutritional Info.
(approx. per serving)

Calories:	150
Fiber(g):	2
Protein(g):	2
Healthy Fats(g):	6
Sodium(mg):	0
Carbs(g):	22

Ingredients

- 1 small banana, sliced
- 1 tbsp dark chocolate chips (melted)
- 1 tsp chopped nuts or coconut (optional)

Instructions

- Place banana slices on a tray lined with parchment paper.
- Drizzle with melted chocolate.
- Sprinkle with nuts or coconut.
- Freeze for at least 1 hour.
- Serve straight from freezer.

Evidence-Based Health Note

Bananas are high in potassium for heart support. Dark chocolate contains antioxidants.

Poached Pears with Walnuts

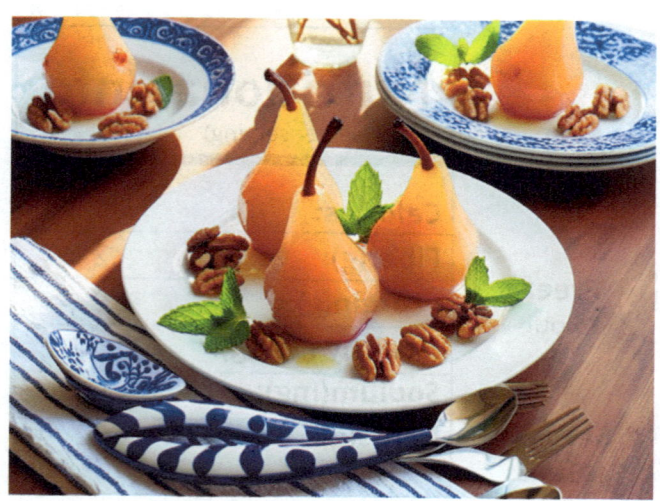

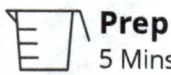
Prep
5 Mins

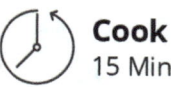
Cook
15 Mins

Serves
½ pear

Nutritional Info.
(approx. per serving)

Calories:	170
Fiber(g):	3
Protein(g):	1
Healthy Fats(g):	5
Sodium(mg):	5
Carbs(g):	26

Ingredients

- 1 small pear, halved and cored
- ½ cup water
- 1 tsp honey
- Dash of cinnamon
- 1 tsp chopped walnuts

Instructions

- In a small saucepan, bring water and honey to a simmer.
- Add pear halves and simmer for 10–15 minutes until soft.
- Remove pears and sprinkle with cinnamon and walnuts.
- Serve warm or chilled.

Evidence-Based Health Note

Pears support digestion and hydration. Walnuts offer omega-3s for brain and heart health.

Ricotta with Berries and Mint

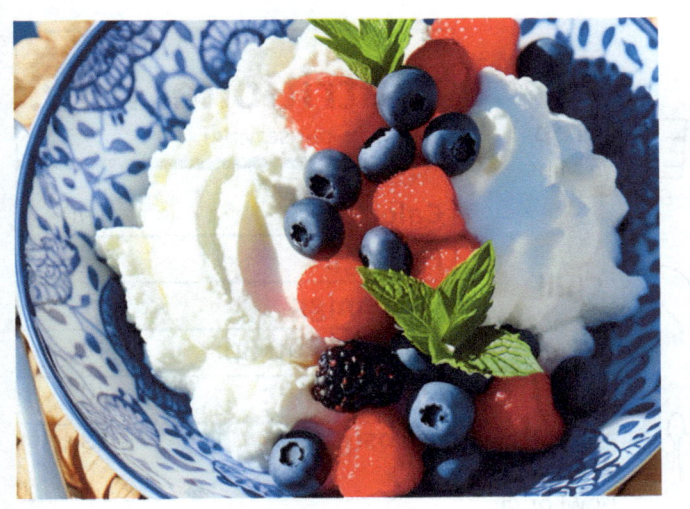

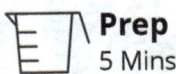 **Prep**
5 Mins

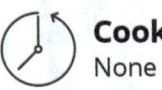 **Cook**
None

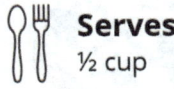 **Serves**
½ cup

Nutritional Info.
(approx. per serving)

Calories:	160
Fiber(g):	2
Protein(g):	6
Healthy Fats(g):	7
Sodium(mg):	50
Carbs(g):	14

Ingredients

- ¼ cup ricotta cheese
- ¼ cup fresh berries
- ½ tsp honey (optional)
- A few chopped mint leaves

Instructions

- Spoon ricotta into a bowl.
- Top with berries and drizzle with honey if using.
- Sprinkle mint over top and serve.

Evidence-Based Health Note

Ricotta provides calcium and protein. Berries are loaded with antioxidants that support brain health.

Chia Pudding with Almond Milk

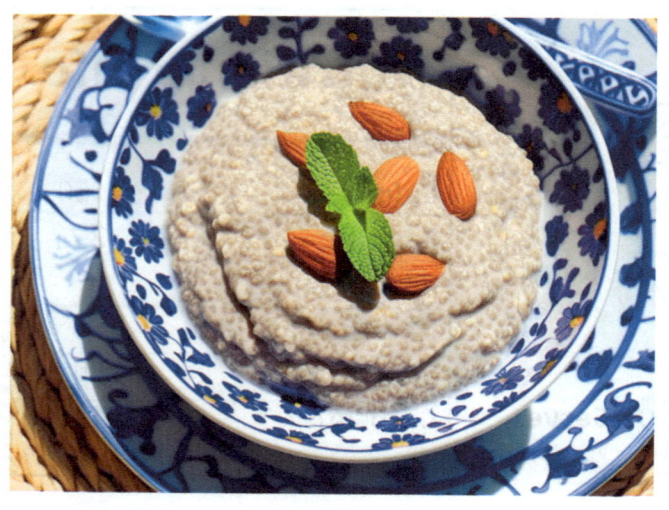

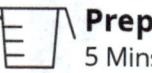
Prep
5 Mins

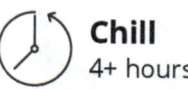
Chill
4+ hours

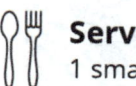
Serves
1 small
bowl or jar

Nutritional Info.
(approx. per serving)

Calories:	190
Fiber(g):	5
Protein(g):	5
Healthy Fats(g):	9
Sodium(mg):	70
Carbs(g):	18

Ingredients

- 2 tbsp chia seeds
- ½ cup unsweetened almond milk
- ½ tsp honey or maple syrup (optional)
- ¼ tsp vanilla extract (optional)
- A few berries or nuts for topping

Instructions

- In a jar or small bowl, combine chia seeds and almond milk.
- Stir well, then let sit for 5 minutes. Stir again to prevent clumping.
- Cover and refrigerate for at least 4 hours or overnight.
- Before serving, stir once more and top with berries or nuts if desired.

Evidence-Based Health Note

Chia seeds are rich in omega-3s and fiber. Almond milk adds calcium and vitamin E.

Refreshing Drinks

Cucumber Mint Water

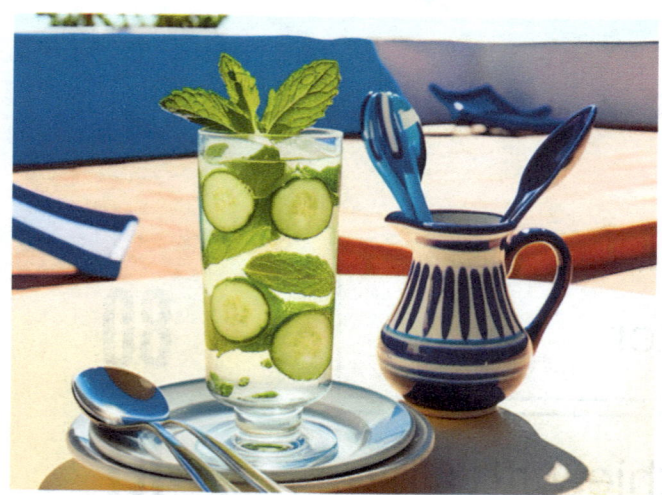

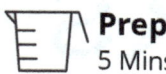 **Prep**
5 Mins

 Chill
30 minutes

Serves
1 glass

Nutritional Info.
(approx. per serving)

Calories:	5
Fiber(g):	0
Protein(g):	0
Healthy Fats(g):	0
Sodium(mg):	5
Carbs(g):	1

Ingredients

- 4–5 slices of cucumber
- 3–4 fresh mint leaves
- 1 cup cold water
- Ice cubes (optional)

Instructions

- Add cucumber slices and mint leaves to a glass or pitcher of cold water.
- Let infuse in the fridge for at least 30 minutes.
- Serve chilled with or without ice.

Evidence-Based Health Note

Cucumber hydrates and soothes digestion. Mint supports gut comfort and freshness.

Berry-Lemon Smoothie with Chia

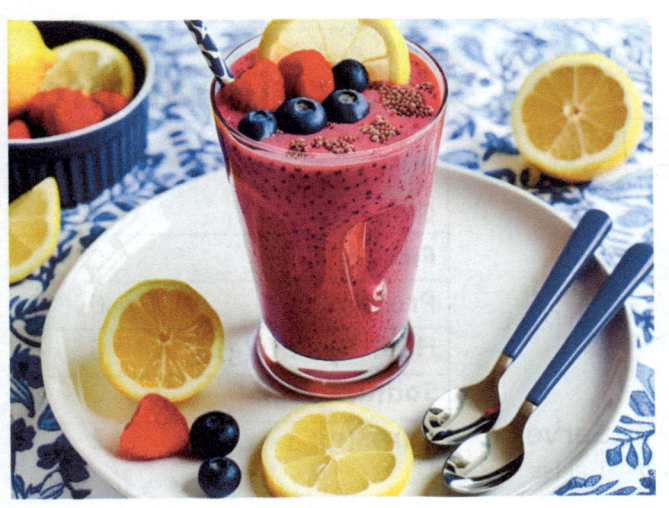

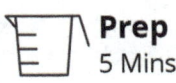 **Prep**
5 Mins

 **Chill**
None

Serves
1 glass

Nutritional Info.	
(approx. per serving)	
Calories:	140
Fiber(g):	4
Protein(g):	3
Healthy Fats(g):	5
Sodium(mg):	25
Carbs(g):	20

Ingredients

- ½ cup mixed berries (fresh or frozen)
- ½ banana
- ¾ cup unsweetened almond milk
- 1 tsp chia seeds
- Juice of ¼ lemon

Instructions

- Add all ingredients to a blender.
- Blend until smooth.
- Pour into a glass and serve immediately.

Evidence-Based Health Note

Berries are rich in antioxidants. Chia seeds provide omega-3s and fiber for heart health.

Orange & Ginger Infused Water

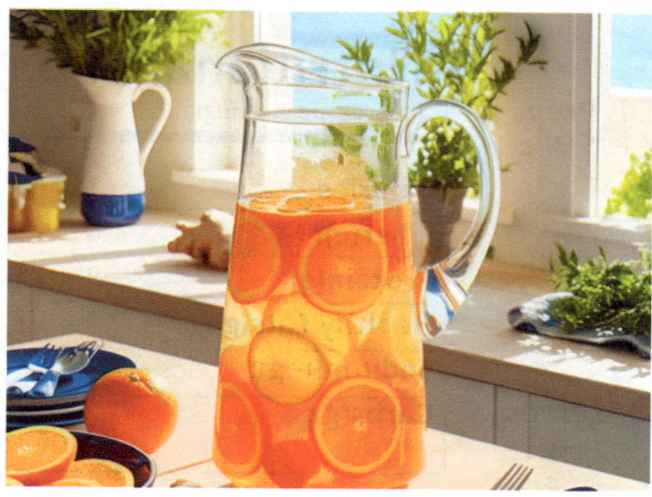

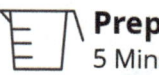

Prep
5 Mins

Chill
30 Mins

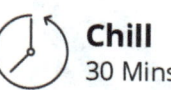

Serves
1 glass

Nutritional Info.	
(approx. per serving)	
Calories:	10
Fiber(g):	0
Protein(g):	0
Healthy Fats(g):	0
Sodium(mg):	0
Carbs(g):	2

Ingredients

- 2–3 orange slices
- 2 thin slices of fresh ginger
- 1 cup cold water
- Ice cubes (optional)

Instructions

- Add orange and ginger to a cup or pitcher of water.
- Let sit in the refrigerator for 30–60 minutes.
- Stir and serve cold.

Evidence-Based Health Note

Oranges supply vitamin C for immune support. Ginger helps reduce inflammation and nausea.

Turmeric Golden Milk (Warm)

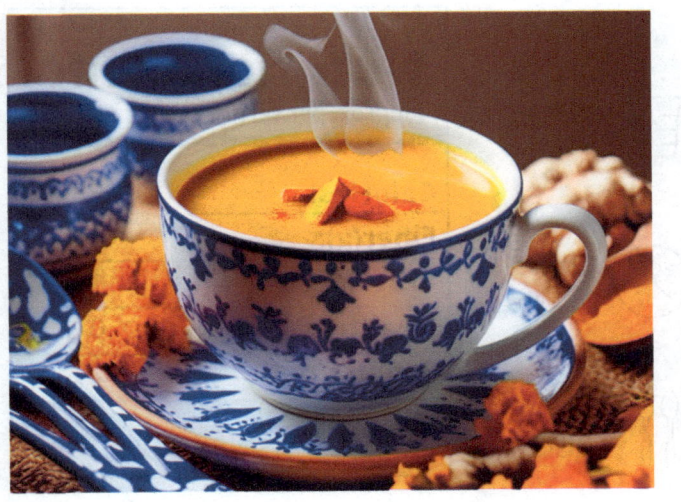

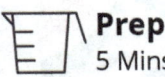 **Prep**
5 Mins

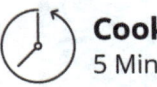 **Cook**
5 Mins

 **Serves**
1 mug

Nutritional Info.	
(approx. per serving)	
Calories:	120
Fiber(g):	1
Protein(g):	4
Healthy Fats(g):	6
Sodium(mg):	60
Carbs(g):	12

Ingredients

- 1 cup unsweetened almond milk
- ¼ tsp ground turmeric
- ⅛ tsp cinnamon
- ½ tsp honey (optional)
- Pinch of black pepper

Instructions

- In a small saucepan, heat almond milk over medium heat.
- Whisk in turmeric, cinnamon, and black pepper.
- Heat gently until warm but not boiling.
- Stir in honey (optional) and serve.

Evidence-Based Health Note

Turmeric has anti-inflammatory properties. Almond milk offers calcium and vitamin E.

Watermelon Basil Refresher

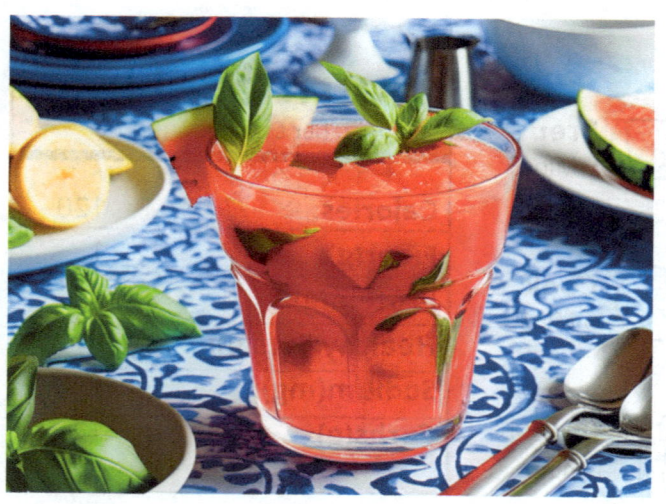

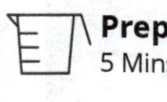

Prep
5 Mins

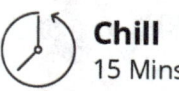

Chill
15 Mins

Serves
1 glass

Nutritional Info.
(approx. per serving)

Calories:	35
Fiber(g):	1
Protein(g):	1
Healthy Fats(g):	0
Sodium(mg):	2
Carbs(g):	8

Ingredients

- 1 cup diced seedless watermelon
- 3–4 fresh basil leaves
- Juice of ½ lime
- ½ cup cold water or ice cubes

Instructions

- Blend watermelon and lime juice until smooth.
- Pour into a glass with basil leaves, tearing them slightly to release aroma.
- Stir and chill for 15 minutes or serve immediately over ice.

Evidence-Based Health Note

Watermelon supports hydration and blood pressure regulation. Basil contains antioxidants.

Bonus
28-Day Meal Plan For Seniors
&
Weekly Shopping Lists

WEEK 1

DAY	BREAKFAST	LUNCH	DINNER
DAY 1	Greek Yogurt Parfait	Chickpea & Cucumber Tabbouleh	Baked Salmon + Cucumber Mint Water
DAY 2	Oatmeal with Chia	Lentil & Roasted Veggie Salad	Roasted Chicken + Frozen Banana Bites
DAY 3	Tomato & Feta Omelet	Tuna & White Bean Salad	Stuffed Bell Peppers + Roasted Chickpeas
DAY 4	Quinoa Bowl	Greek Salad	Vegetable Moussaka + Honey Yogurt
DAY 5	Avocado Toast	Farro Salad	Grilled Shrimp + Berry-Lemon Smoothie
DAY 6	Spinach & Mushroom Wrap	Caprese Salad	Eggplant Parmesan + Baked Apples
DAY 7	Ricotta Toast	Arugula & Orange Salad	Turkey Meatballs + Turmeric Golden Milk

WEEK 2

DAY	BREAKFAST	LUNCH	DINNER
DAY 1	Banana Nut Smoothie	Spiced Chickpea Salad	Tuna-Stuffed Tomatoes + Sun-Dried Tomato Spread
DAY 2	Cottage Cheese Bowl	Roasted Beet & Walnut Salad	Zucchini Noodles + Avocado Dip
DAY 3	Oatmeal with Chia	Greek Salad	Baked Falafel + Tzatziki with Cucumber
DAY 4	Tomato Omelet	Caprese Salad	Grilled Shrimp + Chia Pudding
DAY 5	Ricotta Toast	Farro Salad	Vegetable Moussaka + Stuffed Mini Bell Peppers
DAY 6	Spinach Wrap	White Bean Soup	Eggplant Parmesan + Zucchini Chips
DAY 7	Avocado Toast	Quinoa Bowl	Tuna Tomatoes + Orange Ginger Water

WEEK 3

DAY	BREAKFAST	LUNCH	DINNER
DAY 1	**Greek Yogurt Parfait**	**Beet & Walnut Salad**	**Roasted Chicken + Pistachio Yogurt**
DAY 2	**Oatmeal with Almonds**	**Arugula Salad**	**Stuffed Peppers + Roasted Chickpeas**
DAY 3	**Egg-Lemon Soup**	**Greek Salad**	**Salmon Tapenade + Frozen Banana Bites**
DAY 4	**Cottage Cheese Plate**	**Caprese Salad**	**Vegetable Moussaka + Berry Smoothie**
DAY 5	**Ricotta Toast**	**Spiced Chickpea Salad**	**Zucchini Noodles + Golden Milk**
DAY 6	**Banana Smoothie**	**Tuna Salad**	**Turkey Meatballs + Chia Pudding**
DAY 7	**Tomato Omelet**	**Farro Salad**	**Grilled Shrimp + Cucumber Water**

WEEK 4

DAY	BREAKFAST	LUNCH	DINNER
DAY 1	Avocado Toast	Chickpea & Spinach Stew	Baked Falafel + Orange & Ginger Water
DAY 2	Greek Yogurt Bowl	Quinoa Bowl	Eggplant Parmesan + Sun-Dried Tomato Spread
DAY 3	Spinach Wrap	Tuna & White Bean Salad	Stuffed Peppers + Zucchini Chips
DAY 4	Tomato Omelet	Caprese Salad	Vegetable Moussaka + Poached Pears
DAY 5	Banana Smoothie	Greek Salad	Roasted Chicken + Honey Yogurt
DAY 6	Cottage Cheese Bowl	Beet & Walnut Salad	Zucchini Noodles + Berry-Lemon Smoothie
DAY 7	Oatmeal with Almonds	Lentil Stew	Salmon Tapenade + Chia Pudding

Shopping List Week 1

- [ ] Greek Yogurt
- [ ] Mixed Berries
- [ ] Walnuts
- [ ] Oatmeal
- [ ] Chia Seeds
- [ ] Almonds
- [ ] Avocado
- [ ] Whole-Grain Bread
- [ ] Eggs
- [ ] Tomatoes
- [ ] Feta Cheese
- [ ] Spinach
- [ ] Red Onions
- [ ] Honey

- [ ] Olive Oil
- [ ] Garlic
- [ ] Lemons
- [ ] Rosemary
- [ ] Farro
- [ ] Arugula
- [ ] Oranges
- [ ] Shrimp
- [ ] Capers
- [ ] Eggplant
- [ ] Turkey
- [ ] Cherry Tomatoes
- [ ] Dark Chocolate
- [ ] Pistachios

- [ ] Mushrooms
- [ ] Quinoa
- [ ] Hummus
- [ ] Bell Peppers
- [ ] Salmon
- [ ] Chicken
- [ ] Lentils
- [ ] Cucumber
- [ ] Chickpeas
- [ ] Balsamic Glaze
- [ ] Basil
- [ ] Ricotta
- [ ] Cottage Cheese Bananas
- [ ] Apples

Shopping List Week 2

- [ ] Bananas
- [ ] Flaxseed
- [ ] Beetroot
- [ ] White Beans
- [ ] Zucchini
- [ ] Tahini
- [ ] Mint
- [ ] Oranges
- [ ] Bell Peppers
- [ ] Garlic
- [ ] Tuna

- [ ] Parsley
- [ ] Bulgur
- [ ] Basil
- [ ] Sun-Dried Tomatoes
- [ ] Almonds
- [ ] Ricotta
- [ ] Mixed Greens
- [ ] Sweet Potatoes
- [ ] Paprika
- [ ] Couscous
- [ ] Mini Bell Peppers

- [ ] Avocados
- [ ] Cucumber
- [ ] Hummus
- [ ] Chia Seeds
- [ ] Greek Yogurt
- [ ] Roasted Vegetables Farro
- [ ] Spinach
- [ ] Caprese Ingredients
- [ ] Tomatoes

Shopping List Week 3

- [ ] Oatmeal
- [ ] Almonds
- [ ] Tomato, Parsley
- [ ] Dill
- [ ] Eggs
- [ ] Lemon
- [ ] White Fish
- [ ] Green Beans
- [ ] Barley
- [ ] Kale
- [ ] Greek Yogurt
- [ ] Cucumber
- [ ] Pears
- [ ] Walnuts
- [ ] Strawberries
- [ ] Mushrooms
- [ ] Turkey
- [ ] Chickpeas
- [ ] Zucchini
- [ ] Berries
- [ ] Milk
- [ ] Turmeric
- [ ] Olive Oil
- [ ] Whole Grain Crackers

Shopping List Week 4

- [ ] Spinach
- [ ] Feta
- [ ] Onions
- [ ] Tomatoes
- [ ] Salmon
- [ ] Garlic
- [ ] Red Peppers
- [ ] Celery
- [ ] Whole-Grain Pasta
- [ ] Couscous
- [ ] Capers
- [ ] Oranges
- [ ] Basil
- [ ] Chickpeas
- [ ] Mushrooms
- [ ] Broccoli
- [ ] Zucchini
- [ ] Ricotta
- [ ] Eggplant
- [ ] Cherry Tomatoes
- [ ] Ginger
- [ ] Watermelon

Condition-Based Recipe Guide

(Quick Lookup by Health Goal)

Condition-Based Recipe Guide

Heart Health

- Greek Yogurt Parfait with Berries & Walnuts
- Baked Salmon with Herbs & Olive Tapenade
- Olive Oil Scrambled Eggs with Spinach
- Lentil & Tomato Stew
- Chickpea & Cucumber Tabbouleh
- Roasted Chickpeas
- Farro Salad with Herbs & Lemon
- Olive Tapenade with Whole-Grain Crackers
- Avocado Dip with Lemon & Garlic

Brain Support

- Oatmeal with Chia Seeds and Almonds
- Tuna & White Bean Salad
- Banana Nut Smoothie with Flaxseed
- Roasted Beet & Walnut Salad
- Ricotta with Berries and Mint
- Poached Pears with Walnuts
- Frozen Banana Bites with Dark Chocolate
- Stuffed Bell Peppers with Quinoa & Veggies
- Spinach & Mushroom Breakfast Wrap

Bone Strength

- Honey Yogurt with Toasted Pistachios
- Tomato & Feta Omelet
- Chia Pudding with Almond Milk
- Stuffed Mini Bell Peppers with Feta
- Steamed Broccoli with Lemon & Olive Oil
- Garlic Green Beans with Almonds
- Vegetable Moussaka
- Ricotta Toast with Strawberries & Basil

Condition-Based Recipe Guide

Anti-Inflammatory

- Moroccan Lentil Soup
- Turmeric Golden Milk (Warm)
- Sweet Potato Wedges with Paprika
- Spinach Sautéed with Garlic
- Zucchini Fritters with Dill Yogurt
- Eggplant Parmesan (Baked)
- Grilled Eggplant with Olive Oil & Herbs
- Sun-Dried Tomato & Basil Spread

Digestive Support

- Cucumber Mint Water
- Greek Salad with Olive Oil & Feta
- Chickpea Patties with Yogurt Sauce
- Zucchini Noodles with Pesto & Cherry Tomatoes
- Vegetable Barley Soup
- Couscous with Roasted Vegetables
- Baked Zucchini Chips with Oregano

Immunity & Energy

- Orange & Ginger Infused Water
- Arugula Salad with Orange & Almonds
- Baked Apples with Cinnamon
- Caprese Salad with Balsamic Glaze
- Roasted Chicken with Lemon & Rosemary
- Berry-Lemon Smoothie with Chia
- Watermelon Basil Refresher